Hajer Touil

Repair of facial skin defects

Hajer Touil

Repair of facial skin defects

Overview of facial skin loss repair

ScienciaScripts

Imprint
Any brand names and product names mentioned in this book are subject to trademark, brand or patent protection and are trademarks or registered trademarks of their respective holders. The use of brand names, product names, common names, trade names, product descriptions etc. even without a particular marking in this work is in no way to be construed to mean that such names may be regarded as unrestricted in respect of trademark and brand protection legislation and could thus be used by anyone.

Cover image: www.ingimage.com

This book is a translation from the original published under ISBN 978-620-6-72205-2.

Publisher:
Sciencia Scripts
is a trademark of
Dodo Books Indian Ocean Ltd. and OmniScriptum S.R.L publishing group

120 High Road, East Finchley, London, N2 9ED, United Kingdom
Str. Armeneasca 28/1, office 1, Chisinau MD-2012, Republic of Moldova, Europe
Printed at: see last page
ISBN: 978-620-8-09575-8

OVERVIEW ON

Repair of facial skin defects

Dr Hajer TOUIL

Table of contents

Introduction

In reconstructive surgery, the face is subdivided into six aesthetic units: frontotemporal, orbitopalpebral, nasal, jugal, labial and chin. This subdivision is due to the fact that the facial integument varies in thickness and coloration from one area to another.

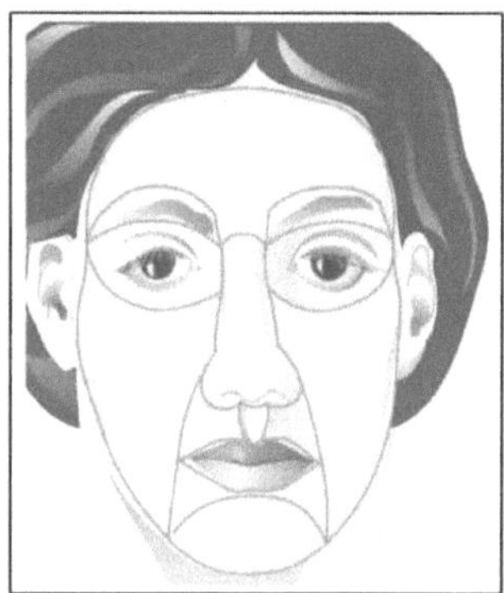

Figure 1: The aesthetic units of the face

This integument is mobilized by the action of the skin muscles, whose resultant forces mark, over time, the lines of tension that become increasingly visible wrinkles with age. Ideally, scars should be aligned parallel to these lines, merging with the folds to avoid maximum tension.

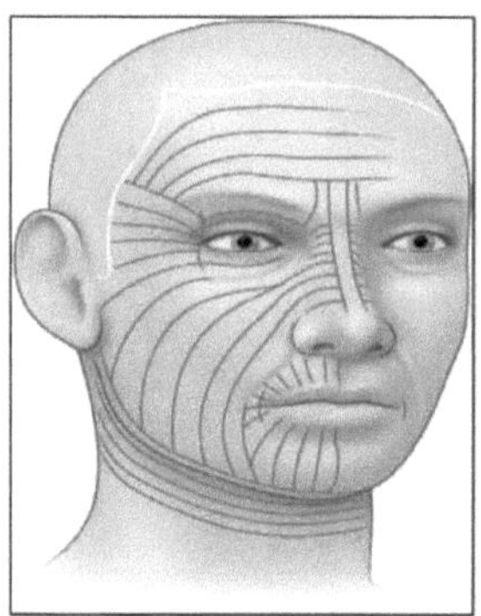

Figure 2: Lines of least voltage on the face

The vascularization of the face and scalp is dense and variable. This explains the wide variety of repair procedures [1].

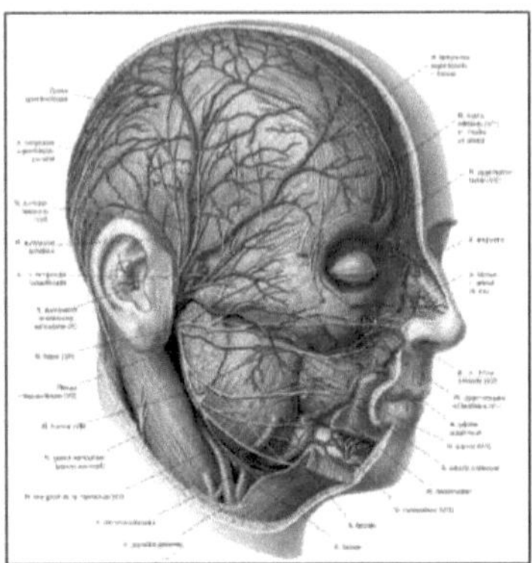

Figure 3: Vessels and nerves of the cephalic extremity

Repair procedures for PDS of the cephalic extremity

Depending on the size and location of the loss of substance (LOS), there are several methods of repair [2,3].

1- Controlled wound healing [4]:

The aim of directed wound healing is to obtain, after an inflammatory phase of detersion, a budding of the subsoil thanks to neo-vascularization and spontaneous epithelialization from the edges of the SDB.

Healing can be achieved by alternating pro-inflammatory fatty dressings, which encourage subsoil budding, and corticosteroid-based anti-inflammatory dressings, which prevent excessive budding. Healing is achieved in 3 to 6 weeks, depending on the size of the SDB.

However, there are a number of impasses to directed wound healing that can block it, particularly in precarious conditions: undernutrition, diabetes, hypoxia, vascular disease, anemia, immune deficiency, etc.

By retracting, the scar reduces its surface area. This often unsightly retraction also risks deforming nearby periorificial areas.

This procedure is indicated for the repair of small SDBs located at a distance from the periorificial areas, notably SDBs on the bridge of the nose, forehead and medial canthus, and in elderly patients.

2- Direct suture [5]:

It must comply with two essential rules:

- Induce a scar in the folds of the face, both at rest and in mimicry.

- It must not cause any deformation of the surrounding areas, particularly peri-orificial areas. It must therefore be carried out without tension or distortion.

Direct suturing takes advantage of the laxity of the facial skin to close SDBs of up to 2 cm.

We distinguish between "donor" areas like the cheek and "non-donor" areas like the nose and ear.

3- Skin grafting [6]:

Tissue taken from a donor site is placed on a well-vascularized recipient site, where it will integrate.

For best success, the donor site should be chosen taking into account the pigmentation, thickness and laxity of the donor area, and the size of the PDS.

The skin is schematically made up of three layers from surface to depth: epidermis, dermis and hypodermis. Thin grafts are distinguished from total skin grafts (TGS) by the thickness of the skin graft. The thinner the graft, the easier it takes, but the less aesthetic it is, and the more its subsoil retracts.

For the face, GPT, which involves the entire thickness of the skin and its appendages, is the most commonly used type of skin graft.

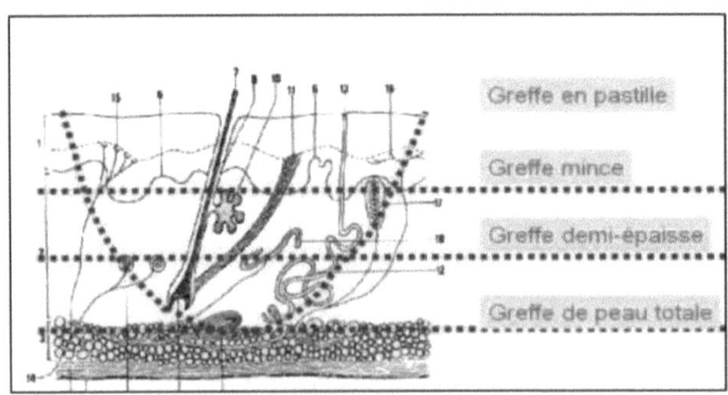

Figure 4: Different types of skin grafts

Optimal conditions must be in place for successful graft intake and survival:

- Gentle graft handling
- Careful haemostasis of the recipient site to avoid any haematoma formation compromising graft uptake
- Immobilization of the graft by a drone with viable, uninfected receptive soil.

3.1- Total skin grafting [7]:

This is a graft that carries the dermis, epidermis and pilosebaceous appendages. The graft, whose size is strictly identical to that of the SDB, is harvested using a fine scalpel, freeing its deep surface of hypodermal fat fragments. The graft is sutured in one plane, without tension.

The most commonly used harvesting sites are: the retroauricular region, where the skin is thinner and of a different color, but which has the advantage of not leaving a scar; the pretragal region; the nasolabial fold; the glabellar region; and the supra-clavicular region, reserved for larger grafts.

GPT can provide satisfactory results in the repair of nasal and labial SDB while respecting the concept of aesthetic units or subunits.

3.2- Skin grafting with a defined thickness [5] :

The thin skin graft brings the epidermis, basal layer and dermal papillae. Its thickness is 1.5 to 2.5 tenths of a millimeter. The graft is easily harvested using a dermatome.

The scalp is the preferred donor site for PDS repair in the various units of the cephalic extremity.

Semi-thick skin grafting involves half to ¾ of the skin's thickness, i.e. an average of 4 to 7 tenths of a millimeter. The dermatome is also used for harvesting.

Although both types of skin graft can adhere to an irregular or poorly septic subsoil, aesthetic results are poor, with retraction, irregularities and dyschromia.

3.3- Compound grafting [5, 8, 9]:

In palpebral or nasal reconstruction, and when the SDB extends beyond the cutaneous plane, a composite graft is indicated. It is either chondro-cutaneous, chondro-mucosal or conjunctivo-cutaneous.

The classic surgical technique begins with preparation of the recipient site. Next, a "template" of the SDB is made. The graft is harvested at the exact size relative to the "template" and the SDB.

A chondro-cutaneous graft harvested from the root of the helix of the external auricle is the reference technique for repairing PDS of the nostril wing. In this case, a small pre-auricular skin flap is used to close the donor site by transposition, without leaving any visible after-effects.

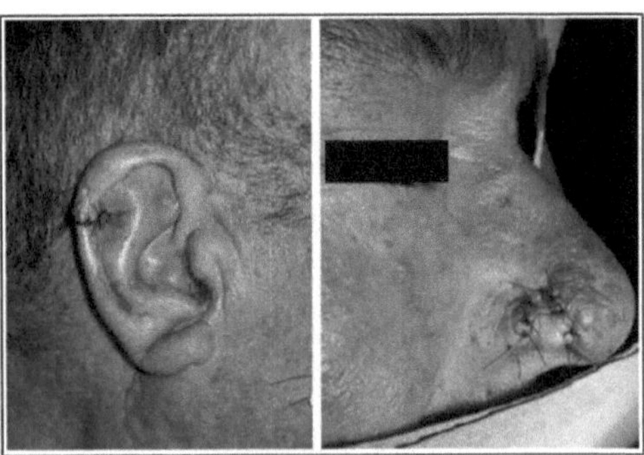

Figure 5: Nostril wing SDB repair using a compound graft

4- Skin flaps:

A flap is a living tissue structure that retains vascularization via a pedicle. The pedicle is kept permanently or temporarily in continuity with the donor site, or immediately anastomosed to vessels close to the recipient site.

There are various classifications of flaps [10].

4.1- Classification of flaps according to vascularization :

➢ ***Random Patern FLap:***

They are vascularized by the deep subdermal plexus. They then survive through these networks, provided that the ratio of length to width does not exceed 1.5. On the face, which is well vascularized, this ratio can be as high as 3 [11].

➢ ***Axial flaps :***

They contain an anatomically designed arteriovenous system. This increases the flap's length-to-width ratio. For flaps with a transient pedicle, the skin paddle of the flap establishes dermal-to-dermal vascular connections with the edges of the SDB over 2-3 weeks. In this way, the pedicle can be severed and the flap weaned [12].

4.2- Classification of flaps according to their mobilization vector :

➢ ***Advancement flaps :***

Using the elasticity of the skin, these flaps combine skin stretching and tissue sliding, enabling direct closure of the PDS without changing the axis [13].

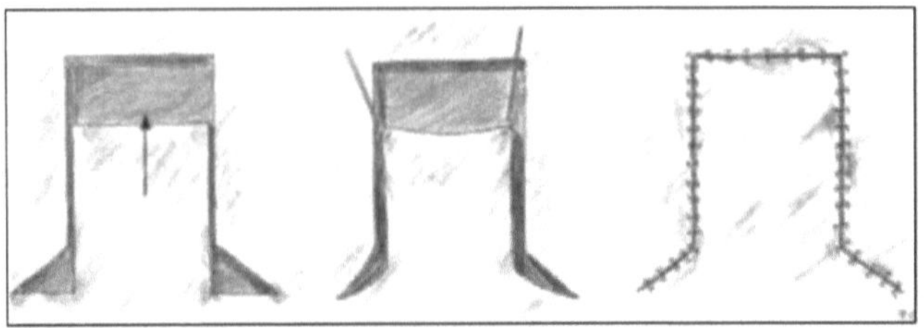

Figure 6: Advancement flap

➢ ***Rotation flaps :***

A rotation flap corresponds schematically to an arc of a circle cut into the extension of the base of a recipient area.

Pure rotation is often insufficient to cover the recipient area. In such cases, an advancement component must be added [12, 13].

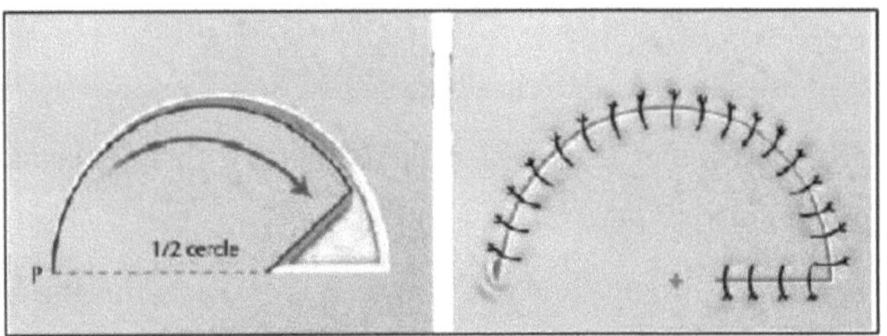

Figure 7: Rotation flap

➢ ***<u>Transposition flaps :</u>***

The principle of transposition is to enable the exchange of a skin flap from a donor site, characterized by its laxity, to fill a PDS located in an area of little or no laxity [12, 13].

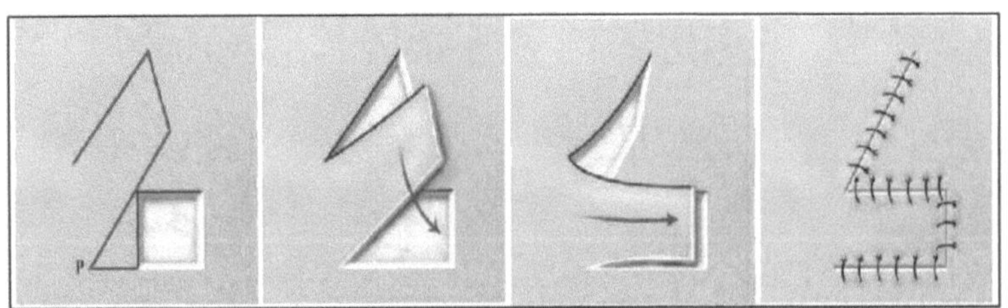

Figure 8: Transposition flap

4.3- Classification of flaps according to location :

- ***Local flaps :***

They consist in moving a fragment of tissue belonging to the same aesthetic unit where the SDB is located, thus having the same coloration and texture characteristics [5].

- ***Locoregional flaps :***

The coating used belongs to an aesthetic unit close to that in which the SDB is located [12].

- ***Remote flaps :***

Pedicled or free, these flaps can be used to provide a significant amount of tissue [14].

5- Skin expansion :

This is an ancient technique used mainly to repair the after-effects of burns.

For facial repair, the skin gain from expansion can be exploited in three ways: local flaps, remote flaps and GPT.

It is the only plastic surgery technique capable of providing skin of normal quality, color and sensitivity [15].

Repairing the PDS of the various aesthetic units

1- Repair of nasal PDS: [16,17]

From an anatomical point of view, Gonzales-Ulloa was the first to speak of aesthetic units of the face, then Burget and Menick defined the concept of aesthetic sub-units of the nose, which are: the dorsum, the lateral face, the tip, the nostril wings, the soft converse triangle and the columella.

Adherence to this concept is currently a fundamental principle for achieving a satisfactory result with minimal scarring.

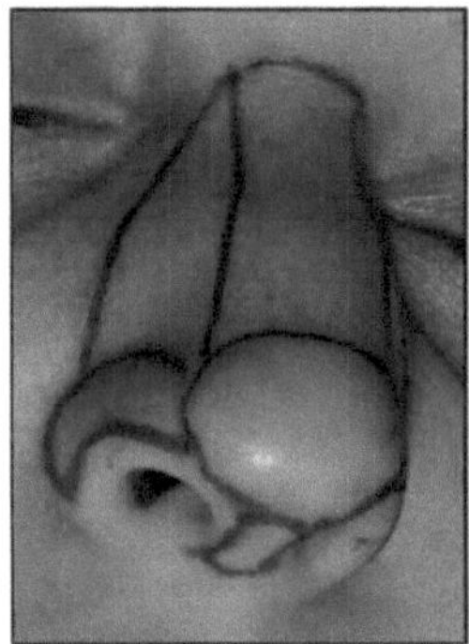

Figure 9: Aesthetic subunits of the nose

1.1- Directed wound healing:

Ideally, it should be used to reconstruct SDB of a few millimeters at the tip of the nose [18].

1.2- Direct suture:

Direct suturing is particularly useful for repairing PDS of up to 1 cm from the dorsum and sometimes from the lateral surfaces [19].

1.3- Skin grafting:

On the middle part of the dorsum of the nose, GPT retract little and give good results, especially in the elderly. The quality is better if the entire dorsum is repaired as a monoblock. Grafting is also satisfactory on the lateral side of the nose.

The donor zone of choice for this topographical indication is essentially the pre-auricular region.

If TPG needs to be very extensive in exceptional indications, such as whole-nose resurfacing, the supra-clavicular region is best suited because of its color.

In addition, composite grafting is a preferred indication for reconstructing transfixing and limited SDB, particularly of the nostril wings. The helix root is the donor site of choice [8, 20, 21].

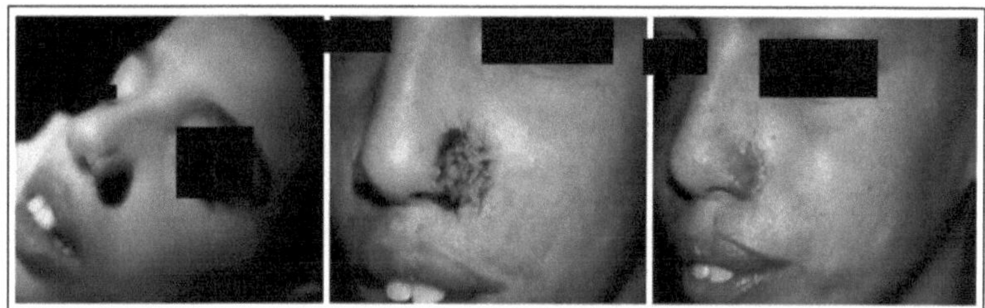

Figure 10: GPT repair of a nasal PDS

1.4- Skin flaps:

1.4.1- Local flaps:

Of all the techniques available, local flaps play a key role.

The upper two-thirds of the nose constitute an important skin reservoir for autoplasty, particularly in the elderly.

Local flaps are used for small SDBs (2 to 3 cm), mainly on the dorsum, sides and tip of the nose.

These flaps are dissected in the rhinoplasty plane, below the muscular plane and above the periosteal and perichondral plane [7].

1.4.1.1- Advancement flaps:

1.4.1.1. a- <u>Rybka island musculocutaneous flap</u> :

It is pedicled on the superior alar artery and based on the lower fibers of the transverse nasal muscle. It is drawn at and above the supra-alar sulcus, with the tip extending into the alo-genial sulcus.

In the anterior two-thirds, the flap is incised right down to the muscle. In the distal third, subcutaneous dissection is sufficient. Closure is performed in VY.

The mobility of this flap is limited, and it is only suitable for SDBs smaller than 15 mm and located at the tip-wing junction but at a distance from the nostril rim [22].

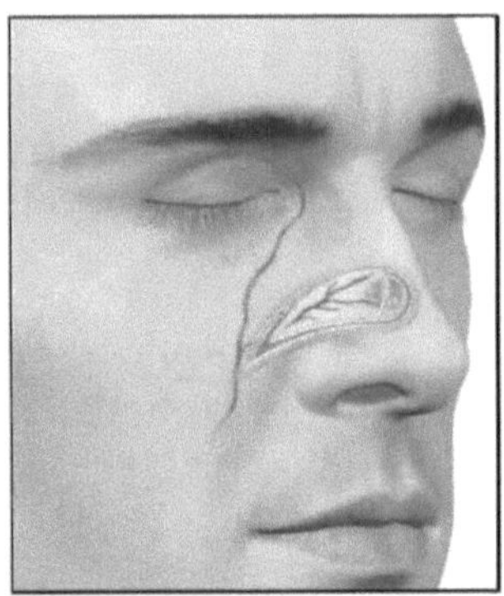

Figure 11: Rybka island flap

1.4.1.1. b- <u>The island advancement flap with subcutaneous pedicle [23,24]</u>:

This flap, also known as the kite flap, is vascularized by hypodermal vessels. It is drawn from the upper edge of the SDB. Its length should be between 1.5 and 2 times the diameter of the SDB.

The triangular advancement skin paddle is freed from its lateral skin attachments down to the subcutaneous plane. Closure is ensured by a VY plasty.

This flap is particularly suitable for reconstruction of the glabellar region and dorsum. The SDB should not exceed 1.5 cm in diameter.

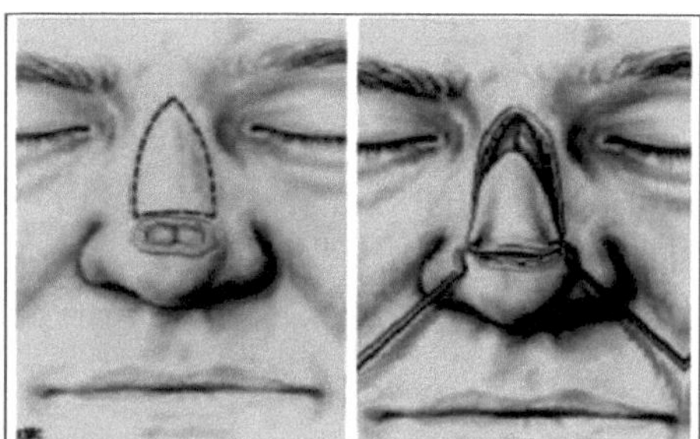

Figure 12: Islet advancement flap for the dorsum of the nose

1.4.1.1. c- <u>The Rintala U-shaped flap</u>:

This is a vertical advancement flap of the dorsum of the nose. It is vascularized by the longitudinal branches of the angular arteries.
The pattern of the flap is drawn on either side of the dorsum at the boundary of the subunits, its length up to twice the width.
Dissection is deep and sub-muscular. The difficulty with this flap is the horizontal suture at the lower part of the nose, due to the difference in thickness between the two edges, which can result in a visible scar.
It is primarily intended for medial dorsal SDBs smaller than 15 mm. It has the advantage of respecting an anatomical subunit: the dorsum, but it raises the tip and leads to closure of the nasofrontal angle [25].

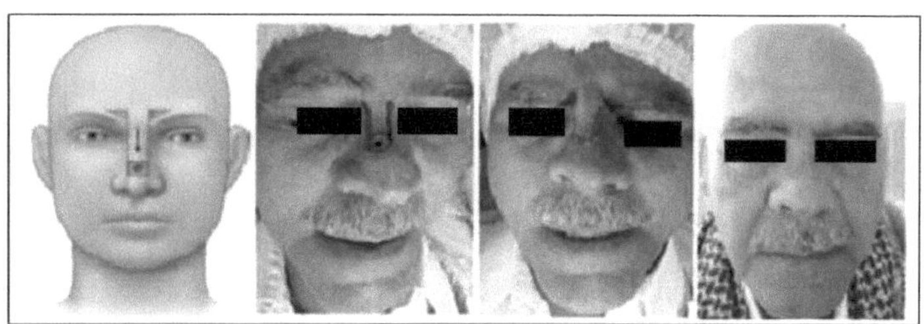

Figure 13: The Rintala flap

1.4.1.1. d- Ono island flap :

This is a fusiform flap, tangential at its base to the PDS, and combining lateral translation with advancement.

This flap, with a subcutaneous pedicle, is indicated for the repair of small latero-nasal PDS [26].

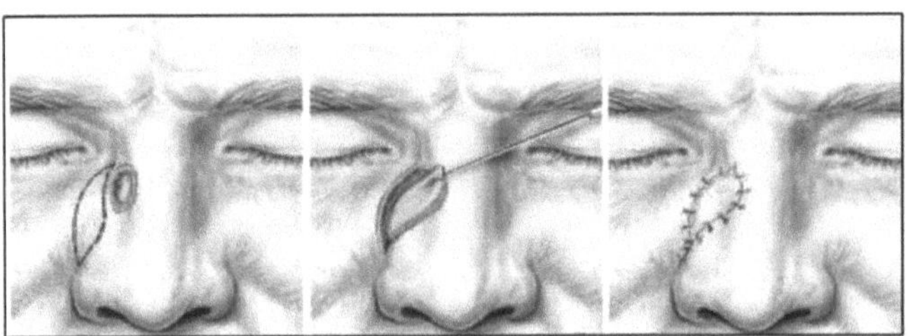

Figure 14: Ono island flap

1.4.1.2- Les lambeauxde transposition :

1.4.1.2. a- The bilobed flap :

This is a double transposition flap. The first lobe should be the size of the SDB, the second lobe half the size and about twice the height, so that it can be closed by simple approximation.

The overall rotation of the flap must be less than 110°, with the rotation of each lobe not exceeding 150°.

This flap is only suitable for SDB of the tip or upper half of the nose measuring 1.5 to 2 cm in diameter [14, 20, 27].

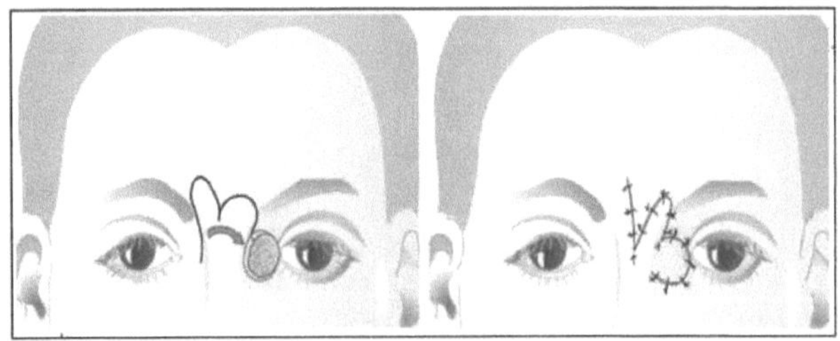

Figure 15: Bilobed flap

*1.4.1.2. b- **The hatchet flap** :*

This is a subcutaneous hinged rotation flap. It is shaped like a small axe, with the "sharp" side tangent to one of the edges of the SDB at one end.

This flap is intended for 0.5 to 1.5 cm SDBs located laterally at the tip of the nose and in the dorsal medial region [28, 29].

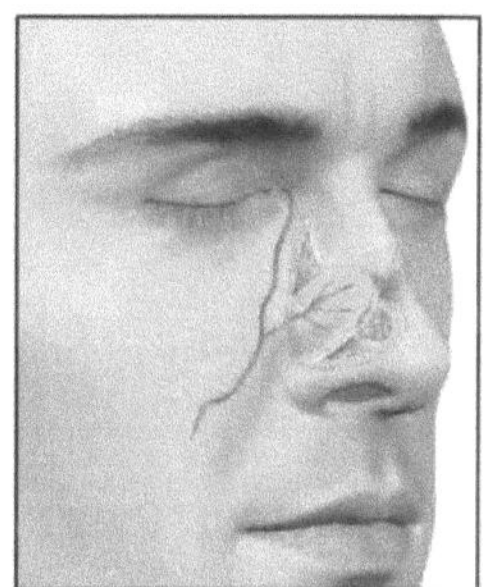

Figure 16: Emmet hatchet flap

A modification to this technique has been reported by transforming the subcutaneous pedicle into a musculocutaneous pedicle, resulting in greater reliability and mobility. As a result, the flap can repair larger SDBs up to 2.5 to 3 cm long.

*1.4.1.2. c- **Dufourmentel LLL flap**:*

LLL plasty is a technique described for the coverage of rhomboidal SDB smaller than 1.5 cm in the vicinity of facial folds and orifices.

Take the bisector of the angle between the extension of the small diagonal and that of one of the sides. Transfer to this line a length equal to one of the sides. We then draw a parallel to the long diagonal of the trapezoid, onto which we transfer another side. In this way, two figures are obtained, which are exchanged after being detached. The donor area is sutured directly.

This flap is reserved for areas where the nasal skin is supple, such as the upper part of the nasal pyramid [30, 31].

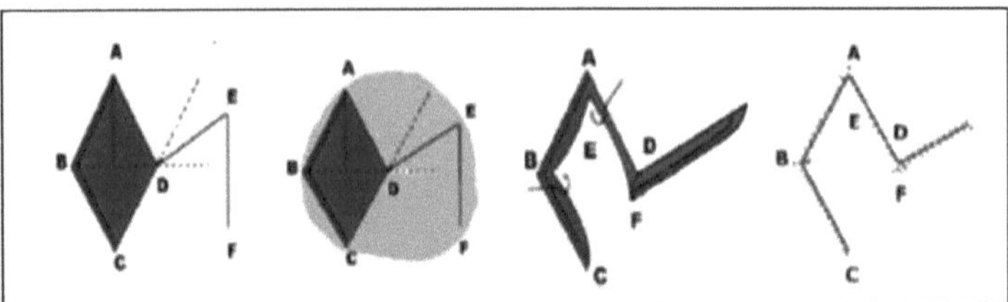

Figure 17: Diagram of the LLL plasty

1.4.1.2. d- __Limberg's rhomboid flap__ :

This unilobed transposition flap features a predominant rotation-transposition movement. It is similar to the LLL flap, but with a different design.

Similarly, this repair procedure is indicated for the preparation of upper nasal rhombic SDBs smaller than 1.5 cm in size [32, 33].

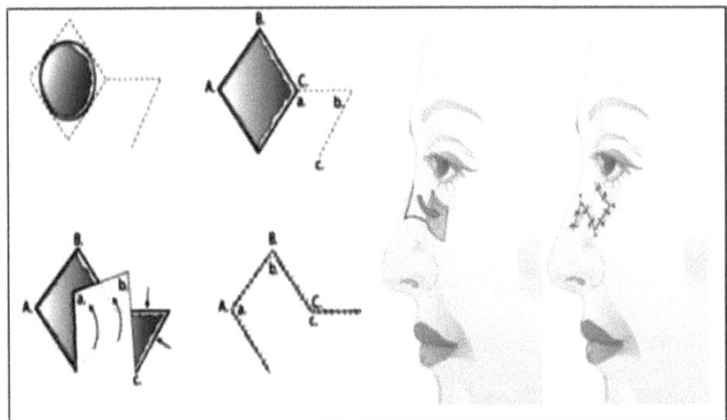

Figure 18: Limberg flap

1.4.1.3- Rotation flaps:

1.4.1.3. *a- **The Rieger naso-glabellar flap :***

This rotation flap is used to repair medial or paramedian nasal tip SDBs that are less than 2 cm in size, while placing the scars at the borders of the nasal aesthetic subunits.

This flap is pedicled onto the angular vessels in the canthal region homolateral to the SDB. It is also vascularized by the broad aponeurotic blade, dependent on the termination of the facial artery.

In the glabellar region, dissection is subcutaneous. Closure is performed in two planes, paying particular attention to the horizontal scar.

This flap is reserved for elderly subjects with good healing and significant skin laxity [22, 34].

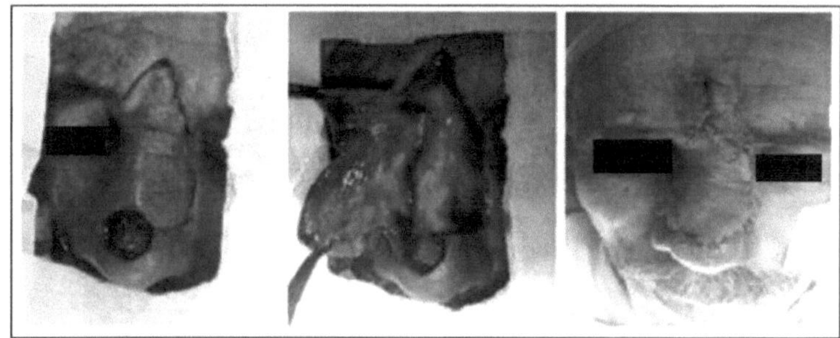

Figure 19: Rieger flap

1.4.1.3. *b-* **Marchac flap :**

Marchac adopted Rieger's technique, pediculizing the flap over the angular vessels on the opposite side to the PDS.

The narrowness of its pedicle allows it to be rotated through 120° to 150°, which is further facilitated by dissection of the muscles of the medial canthal region.

Thus, this flap is indicated for the reconstruction of SDB of the middle part of the nose not exceeding 2cm in major axis [34, 35].

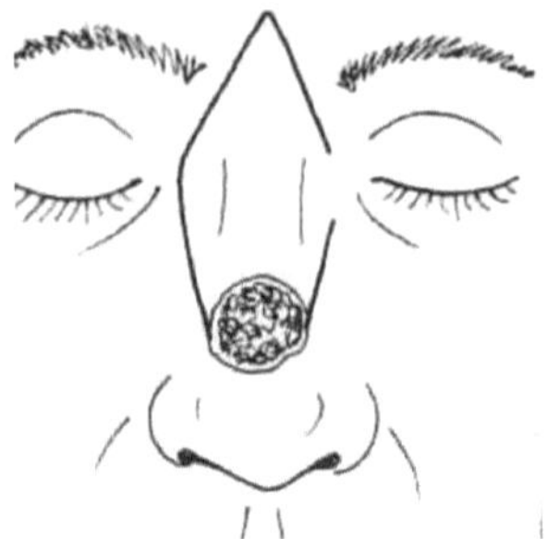

Figure 20: Marchac flap alignment

*1.4.1.3. c- **The glabellar rotation flap**:*

This is an axial flap, fed by the internal canthal vascular pedicle. It is used to cover PDS in the upper part of the dorsum. Dissection is subcutaneous. It results in thick skin at the level of the medial canthus, which must be defatted. In addition, this technique may cause the eyebrows to move closer together.

which can be alleviated by a frontal Z-plasty [36, 37].

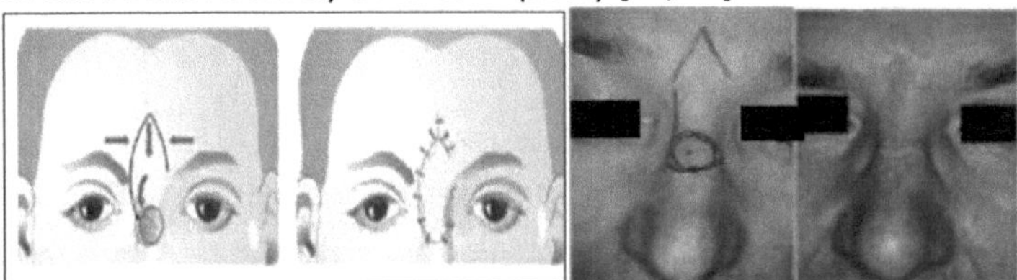

Figure 21: Rotational glabellar flap

1.4.2- Regional flaps:

Local autoplasty becomes insufficient once the size of the SDB exceeds around 2cm. Because of their geographical proximity, the cheek and forehead become preferred donor sites.

1.4.2.1- Nasolabial flaps:

The jugal skin is redundant and generally allows the transfer of large nasolabial flaps.

1.4.2.1. *a- **<u>Préaux superior pedicle nasolabial flap</u>:***

This is a skin-hinged transposition flap, drawn slightly outside the nasolabial and alongeal folds. Its width is identical to or slightly smaller than that of the SDB.

Because of its good vascularization, its width can reach 2 to 2.5 cm and its length 8 to 10 cm, allowing easy reconstruction while maintaining the possibility of closing the donor site without excessive tension and restoring a nasolabial fold.

Dissection is performed in a subcutaneous plane. Intraoperative degreasing of the flap is the most important part of the procedure, and the only way to guarantee a good aesthetic result, as it reduces post-operative lymphedema.

This flap is the reference flap for reconstruction of SDB involving the nostril margin, and folded back on itself, it can be used to repair partial transfixing SDB of the nasal wing. It can also be used to repair SDB of the lateral aspect of the nose or the columella [38, 39, 40].

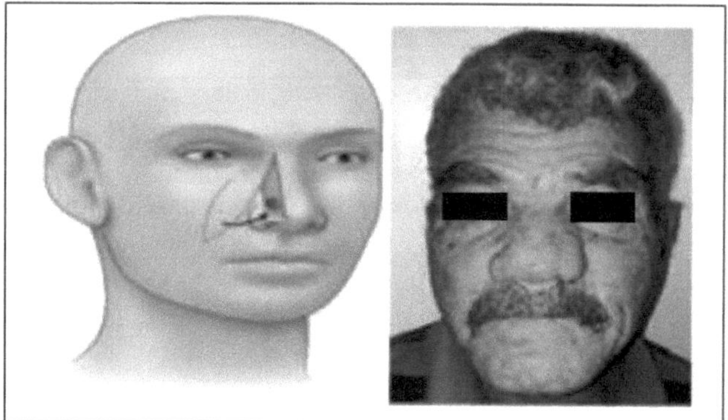

Figure 22: Préaux nasolabial flap

1.4.2.1. *b- **Nasolabial flap with inferior pedicle** :*

This flap is less widely used. It can be used to reconstruct SDB of the columella and lateronasal region [22, 37].

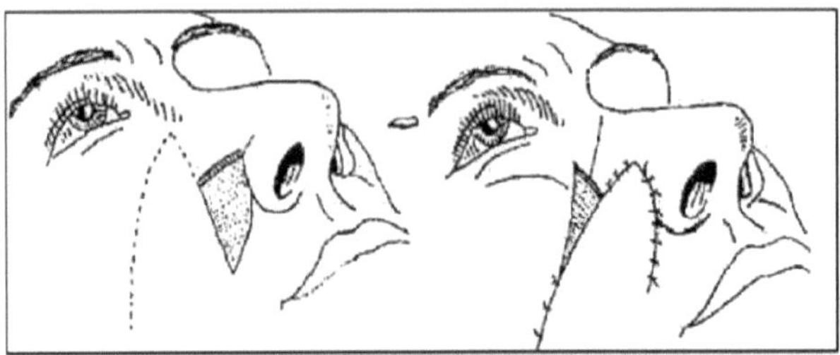

Figure 23: Nasolabial flap with inferior pedicle

1.4.2.1. *c- **Burget nasolabial flap with superior subcutaneous pedicle**:*

This is a transient alo-genic subcutaneous pedicle flap, used for non-transfixing SDB involving more than 50% of the nostril wing. The pattern of the flap, made to measure from the opposite nostril wing, is reproduced just above the nasolabial fold, adding 1 mm to all its dimensions.

The distal end of the flap, which will be sutured to the tip of the nose, is traced at the level of the buccal commissure. Dissection is very shallow at this end, becoming deeper as the nose wing is approached. The pedicle is weaned by the third week. The residual skin of the nose wing is replaced by the maximum portion of the flap, whose retraction accentuates the lobular appearance of the reconstructed wing.

This flap has the advantage of treating the nostril wing in its aesthetic unity, provided that the SDB does not extend above the sub-alar sulcus.

However, partial filling of the nasolabial fold and obliteration of the supra-alar sulcus are virtually constant. When the SDB is close to the nostril rim, scar retraction inevitably results in the free edge of the nostril rising.

To remedy these various imperfections, Burget recommends the use of this plasty combined with a cartilage graft [41, 42, 43].

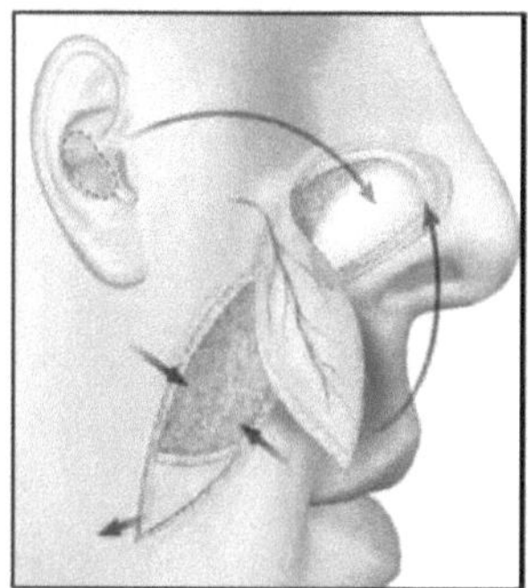

Figure 24: Burget transitional nasolabial flap

1.4.2.1. d- **Subcutaneous nasolabial flap** :

This flap, with a subcutaneous and cellular pedicle, enables the reconstruction of

PDS of the lateral aspect of the nose [35, 44]].

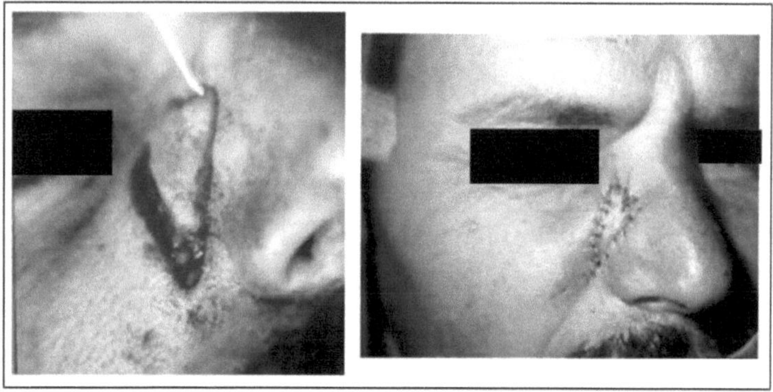

Figure 25: Nasolabial flap with subcutaneous pedicle

1.4.2.1. e- **The nasolabial musculocutaneous island flap** :

This flap is drawn in the nasolabial fold, including the levator muscle of the upper lip and the wing of the nose, this muscle being a true vascular crossroads.

This procedure is indicated for the repair of small SDBs, not exceeding 1cm, of the nostril wing or columella [7].

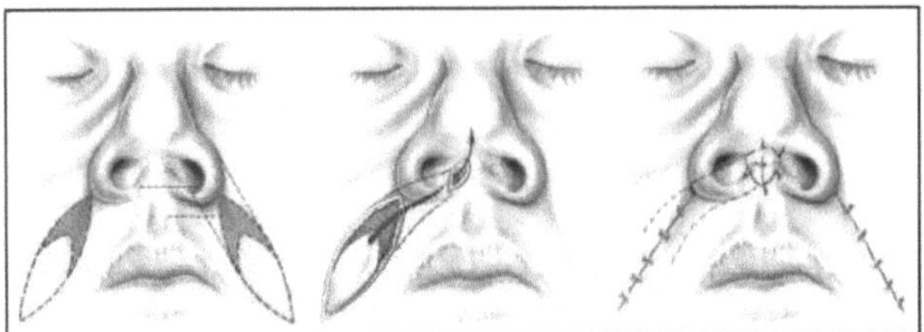

Figure 26: Isolated nasolabial musculocutaneous flaps

1.4.2.1. f- <u>Pers's "in and out flap" turned nasolabial flap</u>:

This flap is pedicled on the superior labial artery, located at its superior-internal end at the level of the aloan groove. It is indicated for the repair of transfixing SDB of the nostril wing margin, extending as far back as the wing groove.

The flap pattern is traced in the nasolabial fold, the median incision is superficial in the fold, the lateral incision is deeper in the cheek.

The detachment takes place in the subcutaneous tissue, superficially over the lower two-thirds, then more deeply, with deep dissection of the pedicle to obtain the necessary mobility.

The flap is then turned around its nasolabial hinge. The upper part is sutured to the mucosal margin of the SDB. The distal part, meticulously defatted, is folded back on itself to reconstitute the nostril margin and the external face of the nostril wing [22, 45, 46].

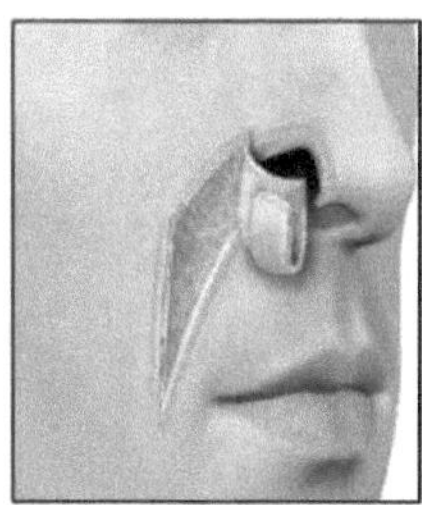

Figure 27: Pers's turned island nasolabial flap

1.4.2.2- Frontal flaps:

The forehead represents the ideal donor site because of the quality, texture and color of its skin, which is close to that of the nose, and its vascular reliability [47].

*1.4.2.2. a- **<u>The paramedian forehead flap</u>** :*

This is the reference flap for all SDB of the nose, whatever the size or location, particularly the tip, wing or columella.

This is a cutaneous, axial flap, centered on a single supra-trochlear artery on the side of the SDB. The design of the skin paddle, based on a pattern of the SDB, may extend beyond the insertion of the hair, particularly if the flap is to reach the columella.

Dissection begins at the top of the skin paddle, and is performed in three different planes. It is strictly subcutaneous at the distal end. In the middle third, it is submuscular and becomes subperiosteal in the proximal part.

Flap weaning is usually performed after three weeks [48, 49, 50].

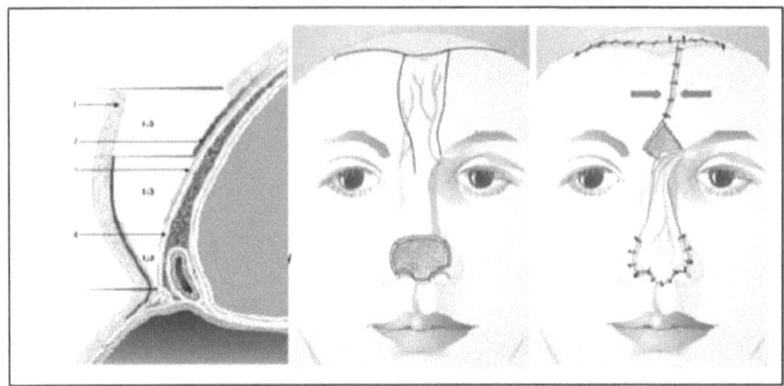

Figure 28: Paramedian forehead flap

1.4.2.2. *b- **The median forehead flap** :*

The medial forehead flap has lost much of its appeal, as it wastes two supra-trochlear arteries and its excessively wide pedicle limits its rotation, making it difficult to reach the lower part of the nose [37, 51].

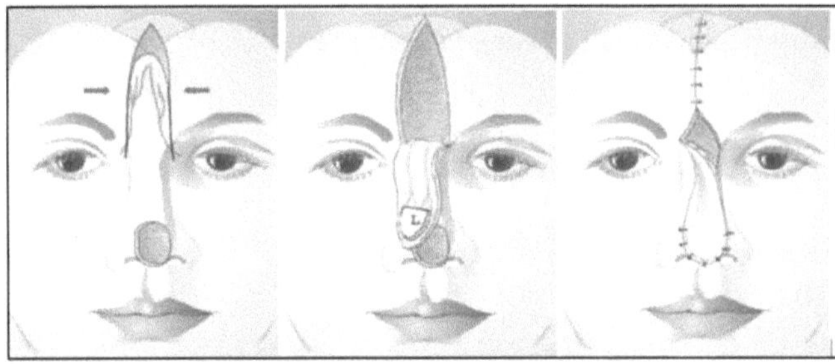

Figure29: Median forehead flap

1.4.2.2. *c- **The oblique forehead flap** :*

The cutaneous palette is drawn at the level of the lateral part of the forehead, with a vascular pedicle that no longer becomes vertical but rather oblique.

Many authors suggest harvesting the frontalis muscle to increase vascular supply.

It is used for people with a small forehead and a low hairline.

It is also indicated when the SDB is low on the nose, particularly at the columella, as this flap has a large radius of action [22, 51].

*1.4.2.2. d- **The island forehead flap with subcutaneous pedicle** :*

This flap is harvested as an island from an internal frontal artery. The incision is made as far as the frontal periosteum in the lower part. Dissection is then performed after the skin separating the SDB from the lower part of the skin paddle has been peeled off. Finally, the flap is tunellised. This flap leaves a minimum of scar and avoids secondary weaning, but in the presence of vascular compression at the level of the tunnel, it presents a greater risk of necrosis [18].

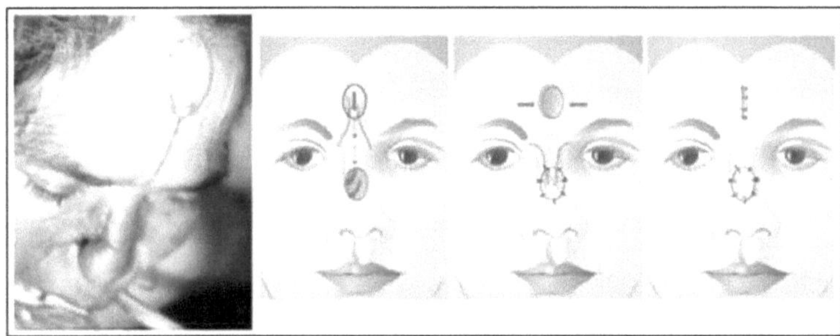

Figure 30: Frontal island flap

*1.4.2.2. e- **Millard's Sea Gull flap**:*

This flap has a distinctive shape with a trifoliate paddle. It is pedicled on a single supra-trochlear artery, and is intended for repair of the outer lining of the apio-columellar complex and wings [26].

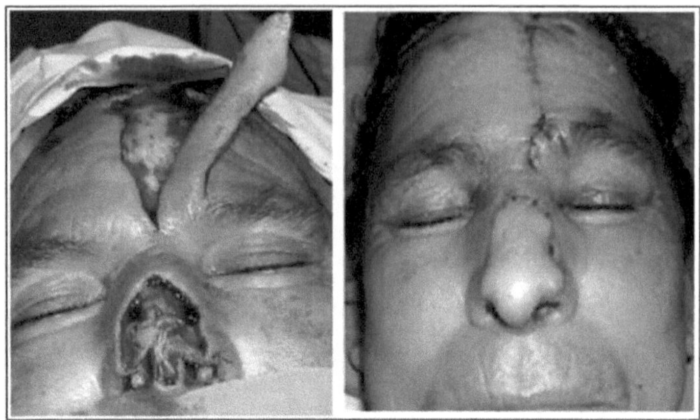

Figure 31: Millard seagull wing flap

*1.4.2.2. f- **Pollet's forked flap**:*

It allows reconstruction of the columella thanks to two lateral extensions drawn on the upper part of the flap, which are spread further apart as the tip protrudes [22].

*1.4.2.2. g- **The converse scalp flap**:*

This flap is used when it is impossible to reconstruct the deep plane with local skin and/or mucosa flaps.

It uses the vascularization of the anterior branch of the contralateral superficial temporal artery, anastomosing with the supra-trochlear arteries. The skin paddle, with its superior pedicle, is approximately 7 to 8 cm wide, depending on the SDB to be repaired. It is drawn on the side opposite the temporal pedicle used. It descends above the preserved eyebrow, with the internal incision 2 or 3 cm outside the midline.

The detachment is performed in front of the preserved forehead muscle, leaving the skin sufficiently supple to harmonize the tip of the nose.

The frontal muscle is incised medially at the same time as the internal incision.

In this way, the incision continues into the scalp from the external incision and joins the usual bicoronal incision path, moving backwards to end behind the auricle. The paddle is then folded in on itself to repair the columella and wings of the nose.

Repair of the donor zone is usually performed at the third-week flap section, using GPT [18].

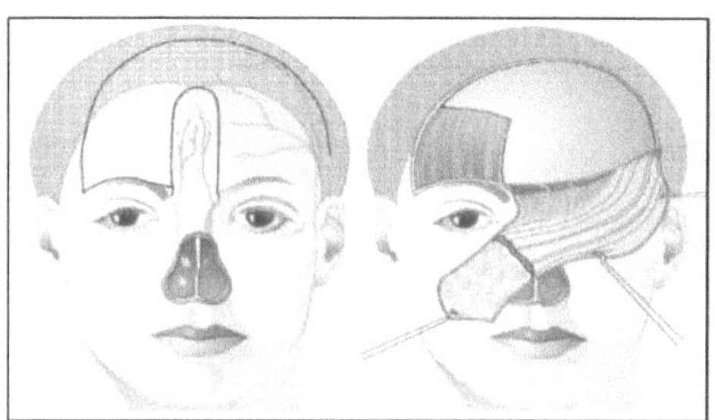

Figure 32: Converse scalp flap

1.4.2.2. h- <u>Gillies "up and down" flap:</u>

This flap is pedicled to the internal and external forehead vessels. The vertical skin paddle is drawn over the contralateral eyebrow. Scarring is significant, minimizing its use [26].

1.4.2.2.i- <u>Median forehead flap with superior pedicle</u> :

This is a medio-frontal flap. Its pedicle is located in the scalp. This flap is used in the repair of distal SDB with a low forehead, or if there is a contraindication to the paramedian forehead flap.

The skin paddle is taken from the middle of the forehead, in the form of a spindle with a vertical axis.

Dissection of the pedicle extends to the root of the helix, so that the flap can reach the columella without difficulty [52, 53].

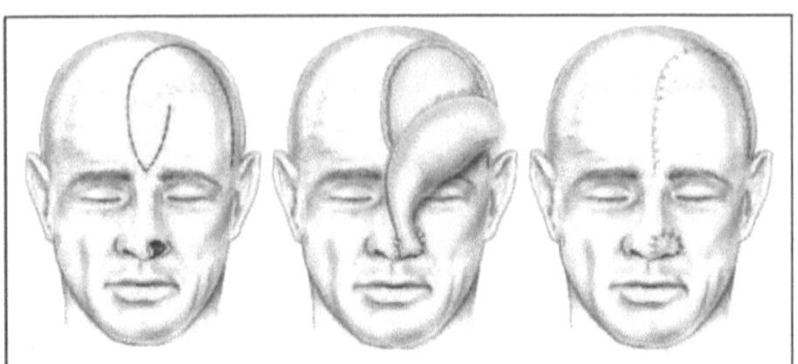

Figure 33: Superior pedicle medial forehead flap

1.4.2.2. *j-* **<u>The Schmid-Meyer supra-arch flap</u> :**

This is a tubulated flap with an internal suprasourcilar pedicle, enabling transposition of temporal skin reinforced with auricular cartilage to the tip of the nose. This is a long and meticulous flap, requiring a minimum of three operative steps, including one for autonomization.

This procedure is intended for transfixing SDB of the nasal wing extending to the tip or columella.

This method has the advantage of providing a reinforced flap, prefabricated to the exact size of the SDB, thus avoiding extra thickness [54].

1.4.2.3- Retro-auricular flaps:

1.4.2.3. a- <u>Washio temporo-retro-auricular flap</u> :

This flap provides auricular skin and cartilage for the reconstruction of transfixing PDS of the nose wing [55].

1.4.2.3. **b- <u>Retroauricular ortichokea flap</u> :**

The ortichochea flap comprises the retroauricular skin, the concha and the skin covering it on the anterior surface.

This is a three-stage technique: first, the retroauricular vessels are sectioned to vascularize the flap on the superficial network. Three weeks later, the flap is transposed to the nose using a pendulum movement on a fronto-parieto-retro-auricular pedicle. Weaning and repositioning are then performed three weeks later [18].

2- Jugal SDB repair:

The cheek is spontaneously less perceptible than the centrofacial regions. In this region, scars should, as far as possible, be placed at the periphery of the jugal unit, or in the direction of the lines of low skin tension [56, 57, 58].

2.1- Direct suture:

It can close SDBs of up to 2cm. To reduce the risk of central depression, particularly in convex areas, it is essential to degrease the spindle corners.

If the axis of the SDB is not in line with the lines of low skin tension, it can be modified with an S-plasty, or even by curving the line. The scar can also be oriented with a Z or W plasty.

The spindle can also be shortened by a V-Y or M-plasty to avoid crossing a peripheral anatomical boundary [59].

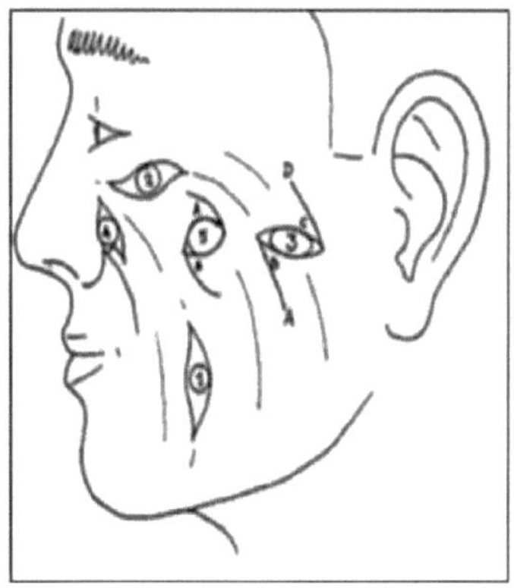

Figure 34: Skin resurfacing; 1: Fusiform resection, 2: S-shaped spindle, 3: Z-shaped resection, 4: Y-V (or M) resection

2.2- Directed wound healing:

Directed healing is often rapidly achieved thanks to the rich vascularity of the jugal tissues. The scar retracts, reducing its surface area, but often remains unsightly. This retraction also risks deforming nearby periorificial areas.

As a result, this procedure is reserved for elderly people in poor general condition and for SDB located at a distance from peri-orificial areas such as the pre-auricular region [60].

In our series, this repair method was used to close a pre-auricular external jugal PDS.

2.3- Skin grafts :

They are often responsible for an unsightly patch effect, especially in internal and/or hairy areas, limiting their use [61].

Cheek skin grafts are therefore reserved for certain indications:

- Coverage of an area at high risk of carcinological recurrence
- Fast coverage for people in poor general condition
- Aesthetic unit coverage, particularly for burn scarring where a local flap is not feasible

2.4- Skin flaps:

2.4.1- Local flaps:

They apply to SDB where fusiform excision risks deforming adjacent areas, or where there is a lack of skin laxity.

2.4.1.1- Transposition flaps:

2.4.1.1. *a- **Dufourmentel and Limberg LLL flaps**:*

The LLL flap is mainly used in the reconstruction of lateral and diamond-shaped jugal SDBs. Incisions are concealed as far as possible in the natural folds of the face [62].

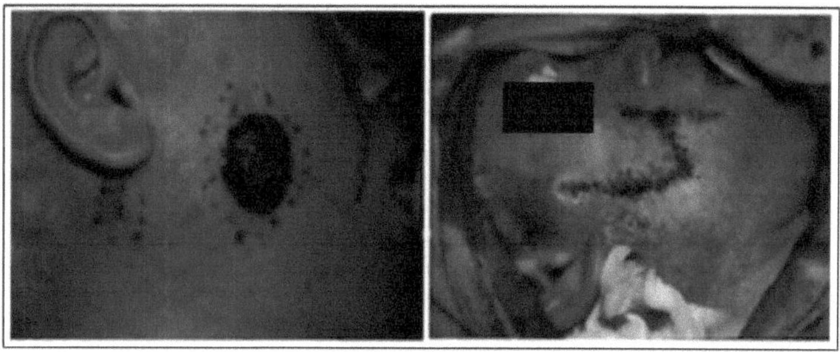

Figure 35: LLL flap

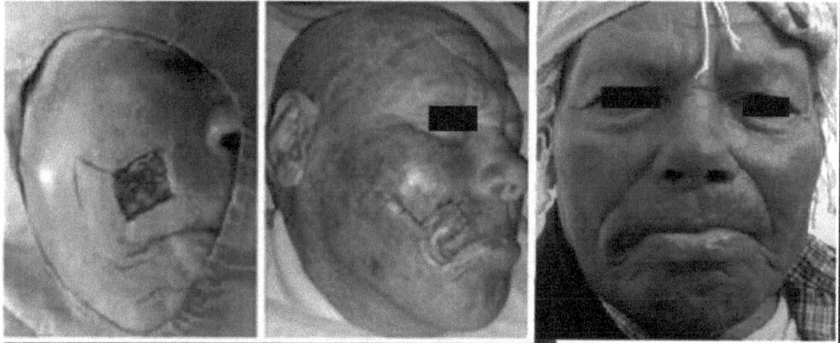

Figure 36: The Limberg flap for a lesion straddling the cheek and lip

2.4.1.1. *b- **The bilobed flap** :*

It enables reconstruction of lateral jugal SDBs using cervical and retroauricular skin laxity. The first flap is used to fill the SDB. The resulting defect is repaired by a second, less wide flap, drawn in the jugal, cervical or retroauricular region depending on the site of the SDB [62, 63].

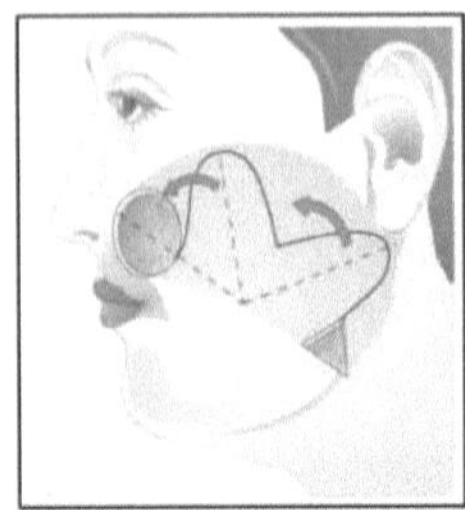

Figure 37: Bilobed flap

2.4.1.2- Advancement and/or rotation flaps:

2.4.1.2. a- <u>The kite flap</u> :

This flap, triangular in shape with a superior base and a subcutaneous pedicle, is particularly indicated for the reconstruction of limited SDB not exceeding 2 cm in the nasolabial region [64].

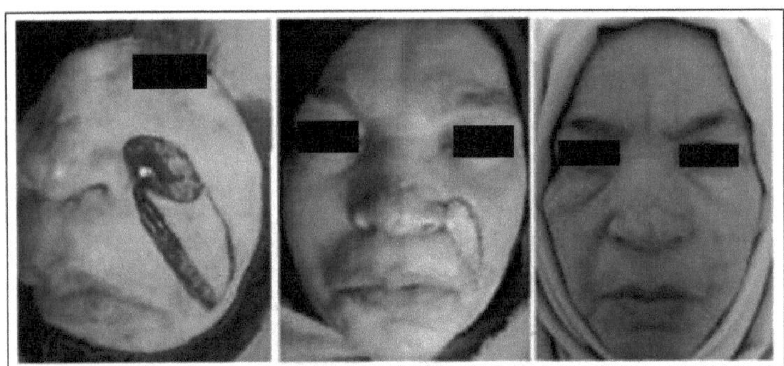

Figure 38: Kite flap

2.4.1.2. b- <u>The temporo-jugal advancement-rotation flap</u> :

Mustardé described the jugal rotation flap for reconstructing the lower eyelid. The same principle can be used to reconstruct moderate SDB located in the upper limits of the jugal unit: zygomatic, suborbital or high latero-nasal.

The course of this flap, vascularized mainly by branches of the facial artery, starts from the superior-external border of the SDB and runs superiorly and posteriorly to join the external canthus. It then becomes arciform with an inferior concavity to reach the temporal region and arrive at the level of the helix.

Dissection is performed in the subcutaneous plane [65, 66, 67].

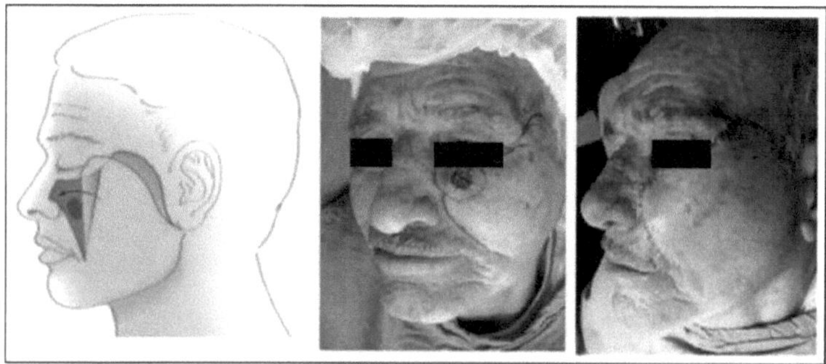

Figure 39: Mustard jugal flap

2.4.2- Locoregional flaps:

They can be used to cover defects larger than 3cm, using localized skin laxity in the cervical and chin/cervical regions.

2.4.2.1- The orbito-naso-genial flap:

It is axially vascularized by the angular artery, giving it a large sampling surface. Its pattern starts medially from the medial canthus and descends medially to the nasolabial fold, then follows the nostril wing and the nasolabial fold. Laterally, the upper limit is a little lower, descending along a curve that is practically parallel to the nasolabial fold. Depending on skin laxity, the maximum dimension is 10 x 5cm.

In terms of jugal reconstruction, this flap is essentially suitable for the reconstruction of internal jugal SDB [68].

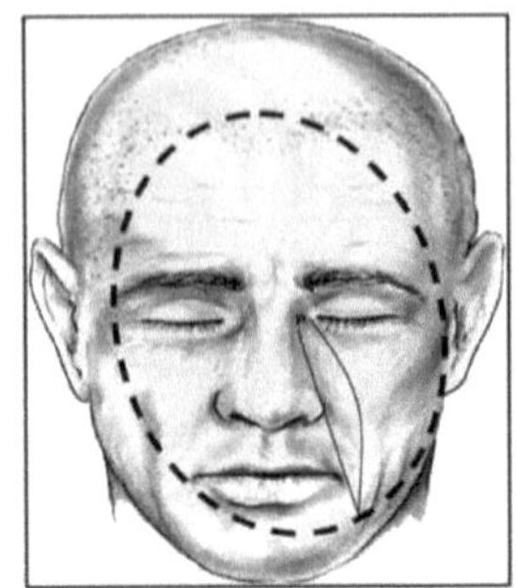

Figure 40: Orbito-naso-genial flap

2.4.2.2- Cervico-facial flaps:

2.4.2.2. a- Starck cervico-facial advancement-rotation flap :

This flap, vascularized by branches of the facial artery, follows the same principle as the Mustardé flap. At the bottom, the incision is C-shaped, ending at submandibular level in the cervical folds.

This procedure is ideally suited to the coverage of superior-internal jugal SDB [64].

2.4.2.2. b- The jugo-cervico-pectoral advancement-rotation flap :

For larger SDB, up to 10 cm, the pectoral skin can also be used.

The line follows the peripheral limits of the jugal unit, bypassing the earlobe, following the scalp line behind the ear, then descending into the cervical region 1 to 2cm behind the lateral edge of the trapezius muscle. It then joins the acromioclavicular joint and follows the deltopectoral groove, ending approximately 3cm above the areola-nipple plate. The dissection plane at face level is subcutaneous, then under the platysma muscle at submandibular level and below the hyoid and pectoral aponeuroses.

The donor site is closed with a VY plasty or skin graft [1].

2.4.2.2. c- Vertical translation cervico-facial flap :

This flap uses the submental cervical skin. It is indicated for the repair of large mediojugal SDB.

The incision passes through the junction of the jugal, latero-nasal, labial-upper and lower aesthetic subunits, and finally the chin.

Dissection is performed along the deep surface of the SMAS. It is extended laterally to end on the vertical line passing through the external canthus [69].

2.4.2.2. d- <u>The submental flap</u> :

This flap makes it possible to use submental skin laxity to reconstruct PDS of the medial region of the cheek in its lower two-thirds. It is an axial flap pedicled on the submental artery.

The upper limit is located just below the mandibular margin. The lower limit is assessed by pinching the skin, so as to be able to close in the first instance.

Dissection is made in contact with the posterior surface of the platysma muscle from the angle of the mandible, avoiding damage to the marginal branch of the facial nerve. The flap is then lifted on the contralateral side, towards the pedicle, always remaining in contact with the posterior surface of the platysma muscle as far as the homolateral digastric muscle. The anterior belly of this muscle is included in the submental flap [70].

2.4.2.3- Retro-auricular flaps:

The retroauricular skin can be transferred as a transposition flap to the cheek [1].

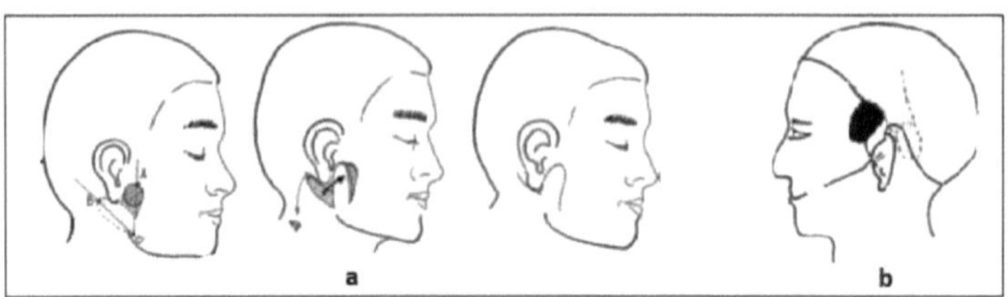

Figure 41: Retro-auricular flaps; a : Retro-auricular transposition flap with inferior pedicle b: Retro-auricular transposition flap with superior pedicle

2.4.2.4- Frontal flaps:

Useful forehead flaps for extensive jugal SDB include the Converse scalp flap, vascularized by the superficial forehead and temporal vessels, which allows the entire skin of a hemifront to be transferred with good vascular safety [71].

2.4.3- Remote flaps :

Often thick, remote flaps are rarely used and are reserved for large SDB.

2.4.3.1- The antebrachial flap:

The antebrachial flap is the most widely used in cervicofacial reconstructive surgery, due to its reliability, ease of harvesting, multiple possibilities for SDB coverage and good cosmetic results. It is a fasciocutaneous flap vascularized by the septocutaneous perforating arteries of the radial pedicle [72].

2.4.3.2- Dorsalis major muscle flap:

This highly reliable flap is characterized by high availability and vascular reliability. It can be harvested in purely muscular or musculocutaneous form, making it possible to reconstruct extensive, cutaneous or mucosal SDB.

The skin paddle can reach 15x25cm. This is a cutaneous, non-hairy paddle, suitable for jugal SDB [2, 72, 73].

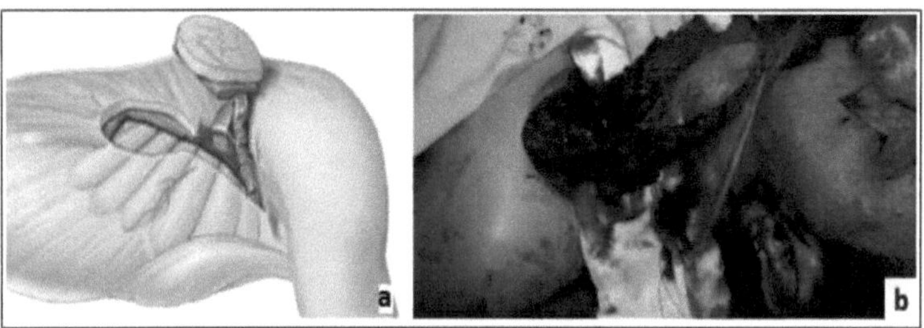

Figure 42: Dorsalis major flap; a : Anatomical basis of the latissimus dorsi flap b: Harvesting of a pedicled latissimus dorsi flap for reconstruction of a jugal SDB

2.4.3.3- The deltopectoral flap :

The deltopectoral flap can cover the lower jugal portion and the parotid region. It is vascularized by perforators from the internal mammary of the second, third and fourth intercostal spaces.

Dissection is performed under the deltoid and pectoral fasciae. Weaning is performed after at least three weeks, and the donor site is grafted [2].

2.4.3.4- The pectoral flap:

It is a reliable flap, but has become less widely used since the introduction of free flaps. Its rotational arc enables it to reach the lower two-thirds of the face.

Functional sequelae are minimal, but aesthetic ones are, particularly in women. In men, hair growth may interfere with the placement of the skin paddle in the mouth [1].

2.5- Skin expansion:

Skin expansion increases the surface area of residual jugal skin or flap donor sites.

This procedure can be used in non-emergency situations, and is best reserved for covering benign lesions or treating after-effects.

The plane in which the expander is placed, at cheek level, is subcutaneous and above the plane of the facial nerve. In the jugal region, the incision is most often located in or at the border of the lesion, or vertically in the pre-auricular region.

The choice of expander shape depends on the area to be covered and the intended flap. If an advancement or transposition flap is planned, a rectangular expander is preferred; on the other hand, if a rotation flap is planned, a round expander is preferred [74].

3- Frontal and temporal SDB repair:

The temple, unlike the forehead, tolerates scars, as it is located in the laterofacial region, not very visible when looking at the subject from the front.

3.3- Controlled wound healing:

Directed healing should not be overlooked when the SDB is of moderate size and at a distance from the eyebrows. Under these conditions, it can produce good aesthetic results, particularly in the temple area.

In a traumatic context, directed healing of non-suturable areas remains, in some cases, the only possible alternative [75].

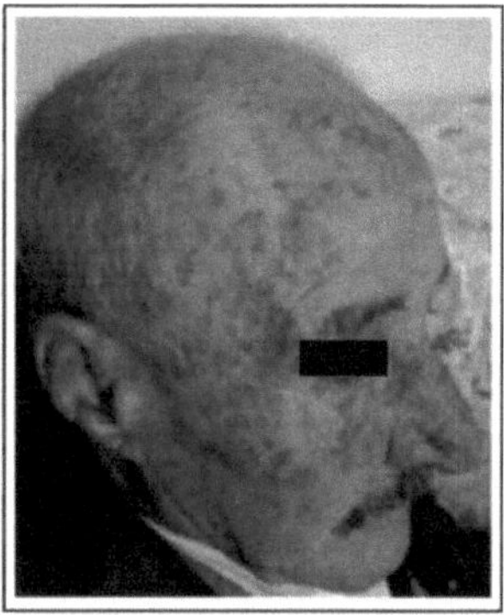

Figure 43: 6-month result of directed healing in the right frontotemporal region

3.4- Direct suture:

This method is used for small SDB and, if possible, at a distance from the eyebrows on the forehead. At the temple, the suture should be oriented from the temple to the external canthus along a radial oblique axis.

On the forehead, the exeresis spindle can exist in several variants. It may be simple, asymmetrical, S-shaped or M-shaped. It is customary to draw this spindle centred on the forehead wrinkles [76].

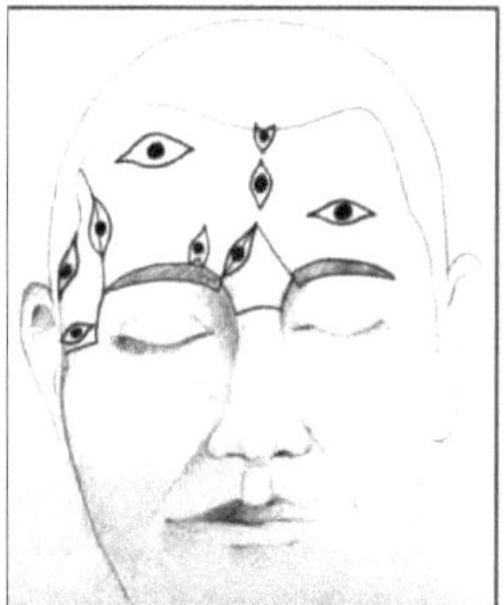

Figure 44: Examples of spindle-shaped excisions: simple, vertical, horizontal, M-shaped

In cases where the lesion is located close to the anterior hairline, especially in patients with high foreheads, it is possible to widen the PDS in the form of a large horizontal spindle to hide the scar at the edge of the scalp.

3.3- Total skin grafting :

For moderate SDB, GPT offers no real advantage over directed wound healing, which often delivers superior aesthetic results.

It can be used on the forehead to accelerate the healing of large PDS and in cases of flap reconstruction. At the temple, the "patch" effect is often moderate, or in any case less visible than at the forehead.

To limit this aspect, it has been proposed to graft the entire frontal and temporal aesthetic units with a total skin graft [77].

3.4- Skin flaps:

The closure must not create asymmetry in the eyebrows, must not descend the hairline, and must not pull on the external canthus.

3.4.1- Local flaps:

3.4.1.1- Advancement flaps:

3.4.1.1. a- H- or U-plasty :

This pure advancement flap, known as random advancement, is classically used on the forehead. It takes advantage of horizontal skin laxity, leaving an H-shaped scar in existing forehead wrinkles. At the temple, results are mediocre. From a technical point of view, it is necessary to take a flap two or three times larger than the SDB. The latter, no larger than 2 cm, is reduced to a rectangle and filled by the two advancement flaps [78].

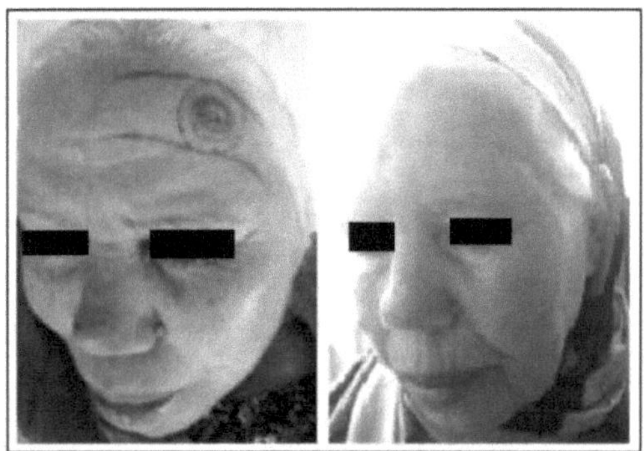

Figure 45: Reconstruction of a frontal PDS with an H-plasty

*3.4.1.1. b- **T-plasty** :*

This is an advancement-rotation flap. It is a pure cutaneous plasty, simple to perform and easily adaptable to all locations and sizes of forehead PDS up to 15 cm.

A horizontal incision is made at the base, superior or inferior, on each side, trying to place it in an expression fold.

A subcutaneous detachment is performed on either side, depending on the PDS. After closure, the result is either a simple T or an inverted T [78].

*3.4.1.1. c- **Frontal island flap with V-Y closure** :*

This is a musculocutaneous advancement flap that uses mainly horizontal laxity and, to a lesser extent, vertical laxity to close the donor area. The flap must therefore be 2.5 or 3 times larger than the side of the SDB.

At the temple level, this flap should be avoided because skin laxity is limited and vascularization is precarious, given that there are few perforators [79, 80].

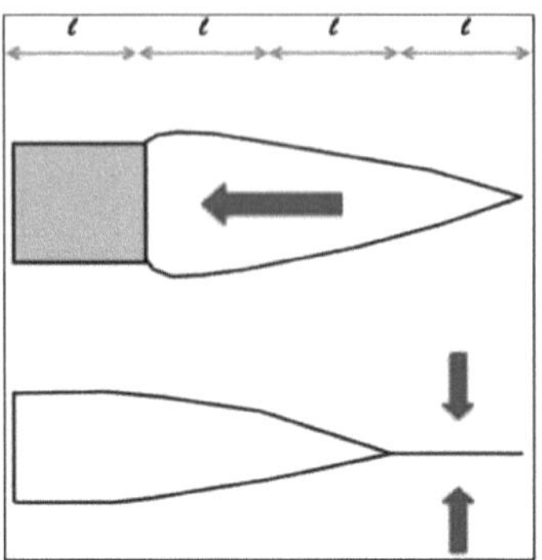

Figure 46: Drawing of an island forehead flap

3.4.1.1. d- <u>Advancement-rotation flap</u> :

This flap, known as an "angled" flap with an inferior pedicle, is used for the temple. It makes use of jugal laxity.

This technique respects the hairline. It places the incision lines at the edge of the scalp for vertical sutures, and in the crow's-feet wrinkles for horizontal sutures. It allows closure of large hairless SDBs of the order of 3 to 4 cm, depending on the patient's age [81].

3.4.1.1. d- <u>Double fronto-temporal advancement flap</u> :

It is also very useful for repairing temporal BDS in the eyebrow-tail region. It adapts to forehead, crow's feet and temporal wrinkles.

It helps conceal sutures in the hairline, on the front edge of the scalp and above the eyebrows.

It also avoids the need to resect excess internal tissue, as it does not extend into the external canthus and upper eyelid [77].

3.4.2- Rotation flaps:

3.4.2. a- <u>The L or AT flap</u> :

The flap is called an L-rotation flap when the skin laxity is used on one side only, or an AT-rotation flap when the skin laxity is used on both sides. These two flaps represent an elegant alternative to H-plasty of the forehead, eliminating one of the two horizontal scars.

They are particularly indicated when the SDB, often triangular in shape, is located close to the eyebrows or scalp, where an H-shaped flap would be much more visible [82, 83].

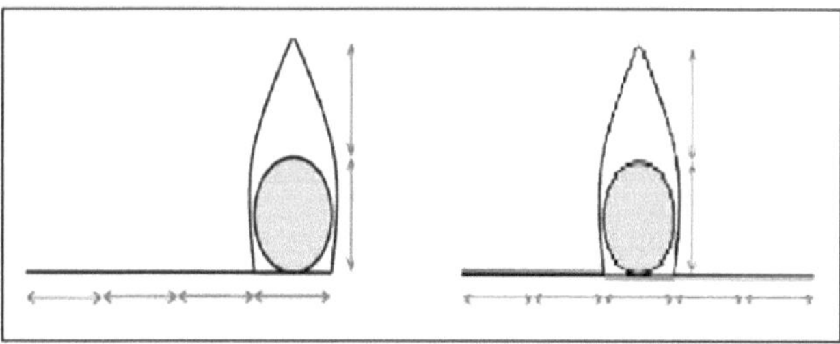

Figure 47: L-shape/AT-shape flap

3.4.2. b- <u>The OZ flap</u> :

This rotation flap is indicated for the repair of round PDS. It recruits skin both horizontally and vertically.

Although scars appear theoretically less well concealed than with an H-flap, the OZ flap remains a good closure technique for the lateral part of the forehead [82].

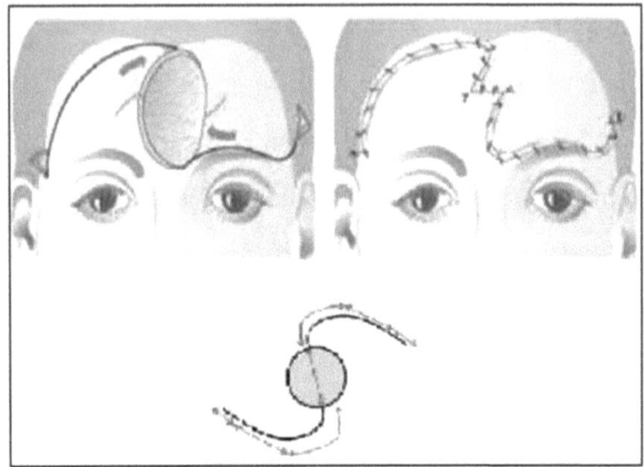

Figure 48: OZ rotation flap

At the temple, try to make the lateral incision at the edge of the scalp, and the medial incision just above the eyebrow or in a supra-brow wrinkle. By taking care to pull more horizontally than vertically, the ascent of the eyebrow remains discreet.

*3.4.2. c- **The fan-shaped rotation flap** :*

A rotation flap can be created, mobilizing all the remaining forehead skin in a fan-shaped fashion. Closure is achieved by lowering the hairline. This procedure is reserved for subjects with a high forehead or after expansion of the forehead skin [77].

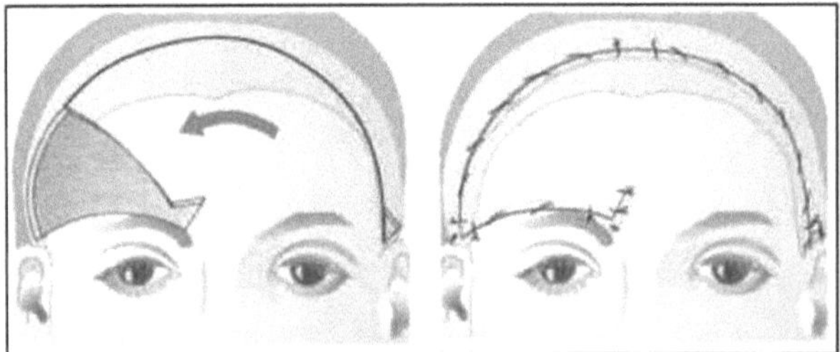

Figure 49: Fan-shaped rotation flap

3.4.2. d- L-shaped temporal flap or temporal "lift" :

These temporal rotation flaps leave a scar on the temple perpendicular to the orbital rim that does not displace the eyebrow, and a hidden scar just at the hairline or sometimes even in the hair [83].

3.4.3- Transposition flaps:

The LLL flap is particularly indicated for SDBs straddling the hairy temporal skin and the glabrous skin. The skin should be taken laterally or posteriorly.

Alternatively, transposition flaps of scalp skin can be used to cover the temple, but avoid bringing the scalp too close to the eyebrows.

The vascularization of these flaps is excellent. Scars are barely visible and define the new demarcation between hairless and hairy skin at the temple [84].

3.5- Skin expansion:

The rigid underlying bone makes the frontal region an ideal site for tissue expansion. The anatomical plane for the placement of expansion prostheses is Merkel's space.

Expansion can sometimes be used to perform large exereses. Expansion of one hemifront allows SDB to be covered from the contralateral hemifront, while directly closing the donor site [85].

4- Palpebral SDB repair:

4.1- Controlled wound healing:

It seems to us that this procedure leads to unjustifiable discomfort for the patient, in addition to the risk of retraction outside the medial canthus, where it can classically be used, for superficial SDB of less than

1cm [86].

4.2- Direct suture:

It is intended for minor, superficial or deep SDB without free edge involvement, and is easier to perform the older the patient.

Sutures that pull vertically on the lower eyelid should be avoided, as they can cause ectropion.

Direct suturing can also be used to repair full-thickness SDBs, typically between one-quarter and one-third the length of the free edge. This is the "Mustardé quarter rule" [87].

4.3- Transplants:

4.3.1- Skin grafts:

The technique used in palpebral surgery is GPT. The graft is then harvested from the contralateral upper eyelid, on and above the palpebral crease.

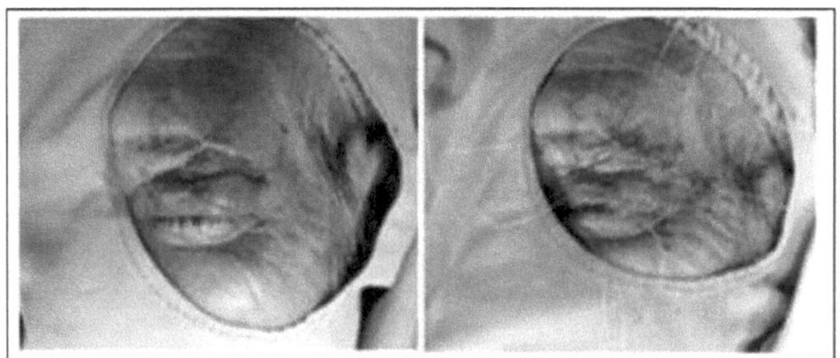

Figure 50: Reconstruction of an upper palpebral PDS with a GPT

At the level of the medial canthus, GPT also gives surprisingly good results for PDS up to 1.5 cm in diameter placed in the axis of the palpebral cleft [88].

3.5.1- Compound grafts :

They are indicated for the reconstruction of transfixing SDBs that protrude beyond the skin, frequently encountered in palpebral tumor pathology.

- **The Hübner tarso-marginal graft:**

This is a simple and reliable technique, enabling extensive and complex palpebral reconstructions to be performed in a single operation. It is suitable for reconstructing palpebral defects ranging from 1/4 to 3/4 of the palpebral length at the free edge [89].

3.5.2- Mucosal grafts:

They are indicated in non-suturable transfixing SDB as a skin flap liner [90].

- **Oral mucosa grafting :**

This graft is taken from the inner surface of the lower lip or the inner surface of the jugal bone. It must systematically be doubled with a flap. Its advantage is greater availability.

- **Mucopalatine graft :**

It has the advantage of providing firm support tissue. Excess tissue should always be harvested because of postoperative retraction.

The donor area is left to heal under controlled conditions with oral care.

3.6- Skin flaps:

3.6.1- Flaps used in lower eyelid reconstruction:

The lower eyelid is more suitable for local flaps. Above all, reconstruction must cover the eyeball and avoid ectropion.

For more extensive full-thickness SDBs, there are two possibilities: combining a skin flap with a mucosal graft, or combining a conjunctival flap with a skin graft or flap.

3.6.1.1- Local flaps [86]:

3.6.1.1.1- Repair of the lower eyelid by itself :

4.4.1.1.1. a- Advancement flaps :

These are musculocutaneous flaps.

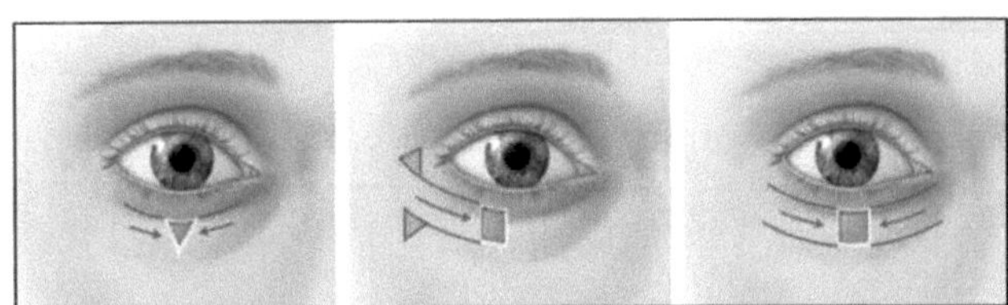

Figure 51: Lower eyelid advancement flaps

- The angled flap:

This is a standard flap, which has the advantage of having only one horizontal incision, thus avoiding "blocking" the lymphatic circulation, resulting in prolonged palpebral edema. The incision is ideally located just below the ciliary line.

It can repair medial PDS of up to 2 cm in elderly patients, thanks to the laxity recruited in the lateral canthal region.

- The T-flap:

This is a variant of the angled flap, where the upper incision extends along the entire length of the eyelid. This flap is particularly suitable for median SDB.

- Other advancement flaps :

They all have their drawbacks and additional, visible incision lines. U-shaped and H-shaped flaps, and the horizontal island flap, are all cited.

4.4.1.1.1. b- *Rotational flaps :*

There may be some rotation in the primary movement of the angled flap. Additional tissue can be added by mobilizing the lateral canthal region with a rotational movement.

4.4.1.1.1. c- *Transposition flaps :*

The rhomboid transposition flap with superior pedicle is rarely used. The medial angle is its preferred region. It must always be oversized.

3.6.1.1.2- Repair of the lower eyelid by the ipsilateral upper eyelid:

4.4.1.1.2. a- *Tripier's bipediculated flap :*

This is a "bridge-shaped" flap. It is harvested above the upper palpebral crease.

It has been described with preservation of the skin pedicles, i.e. by transposing the skin along the entire length of the upper eyelid. Some authors have criticized the narrowness of this technique for its tubulization. Others insist on the need to harvest the skin wide (6 to 10 mm) to guarantee the best aesthetic result.

This procedure is indicated for the repair of SDB occupying more than one-third of the lower eyelid.

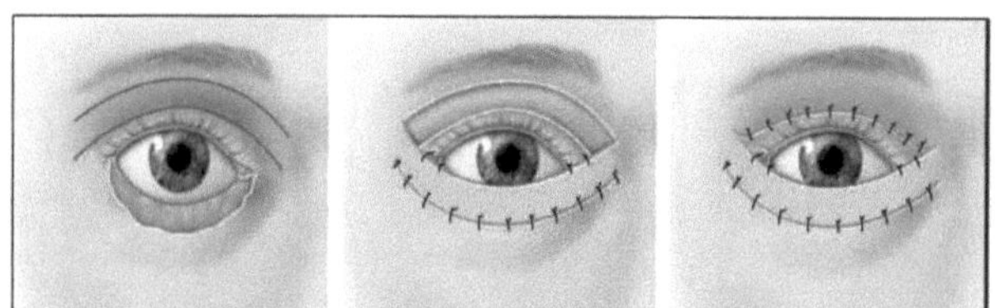

Figure 52: Tripier bipediculated flap

4.4.1.1.2. b- *Unipediculated upper palpebral skin flap :*

This transposition flap, which removes the upper palpebral skin above the palpebral fold, has an external or internal pedicle. Its height and length are determined according to the PDS. It is a reliable flap, although its tip often suffers in the first few days postoperatively.

3.6.1.2- Locoregional flaps [6, 91]:

3.6.1.2.1- Temporal and/or jugal skin flaps:

4.4.1.2.1. *a-* ***Mustardé temporo-jugal rotation-avancement flap*** *:*

This is the technique of choice for reconstruction of large SDBs of the lower eyelid. This large flap mobilizes the jugal and infra-temporal skin. The incision line is placed 1 mm from the free edge of the lower eyelid and must extend well above the external canthal line to avoid tegumental ptosis and secondary ectropion.

The flap is detached behind the orbicularis in the palpebral portion and subcutaneously outside the external orbital process.

This is a thick flap that requires suturing of the deep plane to the temporal region and to the periosteum of the inferior and lateral orbital rims.

To avoid the appearance of round eyes and ectropion, a nasal chondromucosal or palatal fibromucosa graft is placed for reconstruction of the tarso-conjunctival plane [92].

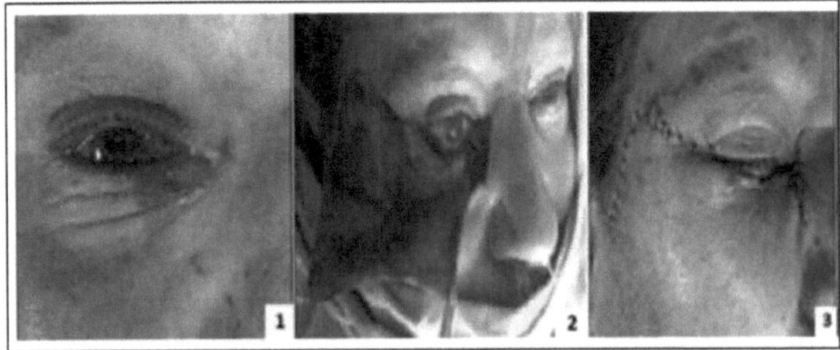

Figure 53: Mustardé temporo-jugal rotation-avancement flap

1: Ulcerated lesion occupying the inner third of the eyelid 2: Lifting of a Mustardé temporo-jugal flap 3 and 4: Immediate postoperative appearance and at 6 months' follow-up

4.4.1.2.1. b- Tenzel technique :

This technique uses a semicircular rotational musculocutaneous flap with an inferior pedicle, whose outer limits lie in the extension of the eyebrow. This flap folds less smoothly than the Mustardé temporo-jugal flap. It is therefore used in cases of rather external deficiency occupying 40% to 60% of the palpebral length [93, 94].

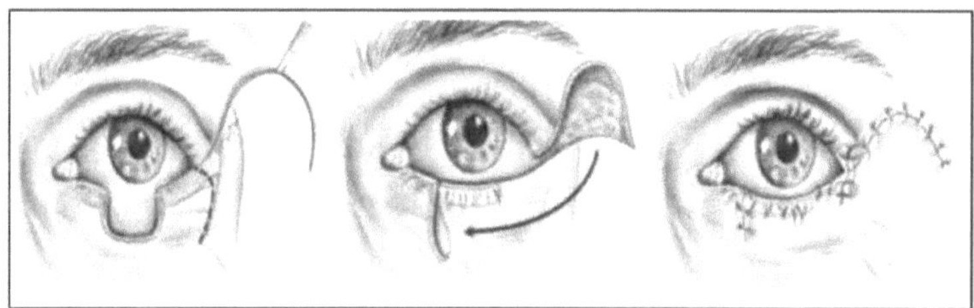

Figure 54: Tenzel repair process

4.4.1.2.1. c- Tessier orbital-nasogenic flap :

Already described, this flap may be suitable for total inferior blepharopoiesis, in which case its tip must reach the external canthus or even extend beyond it.

Its thickness means that it needs to be anchored to the external orbital periosteum in total reconstructions of SDB extending beyond the skin plane [68, 95].

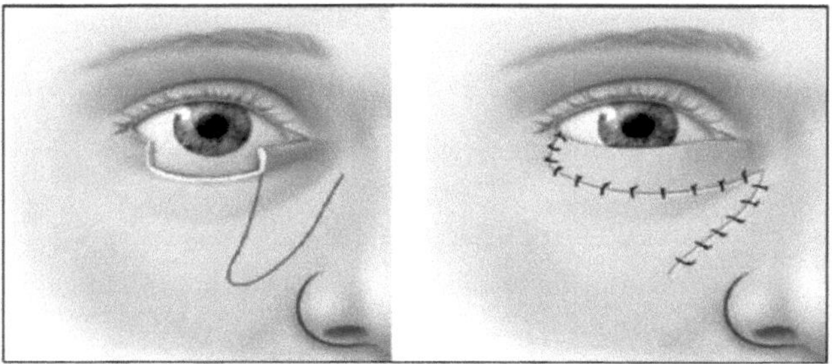

Figure 55: Tessier orbito-nasogeal flap

3.6.1.2.2- Cutaneous flaps of frontal origin :

The median or paramedian forehead flap helps to counteract gravity, but has major drawbacks: the color and texture of the forehead skin is too thick and rigid compared to the palpebral skin.

Some authors have suggested using only the frontal muscle and fascia in the form of fascio-muscular flaps to avoid excessive thickness.

These flaps provide support for mucosal and skin grafts and appear to be useful in inferior total blepharopoiesis [93].

3.6.2- Flaps used in upper eyelid SDB repair:

The upper eyelid is less affected by tumors, but its reconstruction is much more delicate. The surgeon is faced with two imperatives: on the one hand, to ensure good coverage of the eyeball, and on the other, to ensure good palpebral mobility thanks to a fine, toned eyelid.

3.6.2.1- Local flaps using residual palpebral skin:

4.4.2.1. a- The glide flap :

The upper palpebral skin is unwound to form a gliding flap, by means of a wide skin detachment. The skin then descends vertically to cover the SDB [96].

4.4.2.1. b- Tripier's bipediculated flap :

This musculocutaneous flap is used to cover the cutaneous plane of the free edge of the upper eyelid in its pretarsal portion. The donor area is closed by a GPT or a suprasuperciliary flap [97].

4.4.2.1. c- The unipediculated musculocutaneous flap :

This flap, with internal or external pedicle, is limited in length as it is exposed to distal necrosis, and limited in width, hence its tendency to tubulization [98].

3.6.2.2- Locoregional flaps:

The lower eyelid, frontal region and pre-auricular region can be donor sites.

4.4.2.2. a- <u>The Fricke suprasuperciliary flap</u> :

This is a forehead flap with an inferolateral pedicle, traced horizontally above the eyebrow. It has no axial vascularization and requires one or more prior autonomizations, especially in smokers.

It tends to thicken and shrink in on itself during the various empowerment phases. For this reason, its width should be greater than the height of the PDS, and its length should be greater than the height of the PDS, as distal distress may occur during insertion [90, 94].

4.4.2.2. b- <u>Retrograde flow islet flap</u> :

This technique, described by a number of authors, makes it possible to supply integuments vascularized by retrograde-flow superficial temporal vessels to the upper eyelids and external canthus [98].

4.4.2.2. c- <u>Flaps using the lower eyelid</u> :

These techniques are indicated for the reconstruction of transfixing SDB, frequently encountered in palpebral tumor pathology.

> <u>The Esser-Mustardé technique</u> :

It uses a full-thickness inferior palpebral flap, vascularized by the ciliary margin artery. The harvested palpebral fragment is rotated 180° in the frontal plane and remains attached to the donor site by its pedicle for 15 days [98].

For SDB of half the upper eyelid or less, only a quarter of the lower eyelid is required. The pedicle must be located in the middle of the loss of substance. The flap should be traced on the temporal side of this landmark. The donor site is closed directly by full-thickness suture of the lower eyelid.

For total SDB of the upper eyelid, it is necessary to remove more than a quarter of the lower eyelid.

The residual inferior palpebral PDS is then closed by a temporo-jugal flap in a second stage, on postoperative day 15ème .

Some authors, on the other hand, place the pedicle on the outer edge of the flap at the end of a temporo-jugal flap. In these cases, reconstruction is performed in a single stage.

> **The Cutler-Beard flap :**

Although it presents many difficulties, it can be used for partial deficits, but especially for complete deficits of the upper eyelid.

This is an ascension flap from the lower to the upper eyelid through a subtarsal incision, preserving the free border of the lower eyelid.

The incision is located 5 mm below the free edge of the lower eyelid, is transfixing, and the flap is U-shaped with an inferior pedicle. It passes behind the free border of the lower eyelid. The flap is sutured in two or three planes to the edges of the upper palpebral SDB.

This flap should be left in place for at least 6 weeks before trimming the pedicle. It is prudent to leave an excess of conjunctiva at the free edge during separation [99].

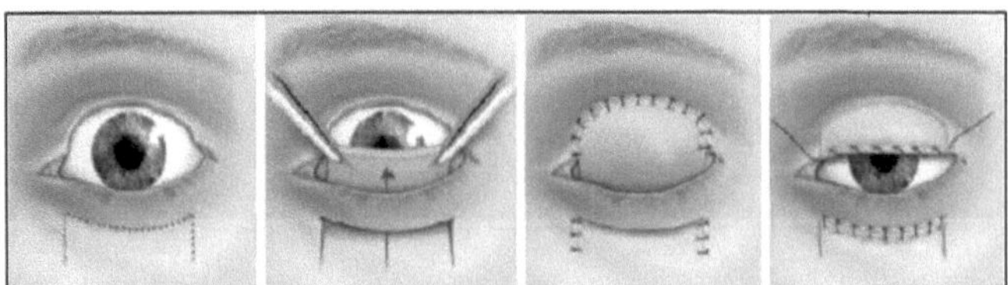

Figure 56: Technique for repairing the upper eyelid with a Cutler-Beard flap

3.6.3- Flaps used in the repair of PDS of the medial canthus:

Reconstructing PDS in this region is complex.

The choice of a reconstruction technique depends on the following factors:

- the medial palpebral ligament: is it continuous?
- Is the lacrimal duct damaged?

For cutaneous SDB, glabellar and forehead flaps are the most commonly used. The deep surface of the flap must be docked to the periosteum of the orbito-nasal angle, so that the flap lies harmoniously [26].

3.6.4- Flaps used in the repair of PDS of the external canthus :

Rotation flaps, which remove the skin and orbicularis muscle from the upper eyelid, close most superficial SDBs.

An LLL-type line, with an external pedicle, is particularly suitable for harvesting excess upper palpebral skin.

For complex SDPs, you need :

- reconstruct conjunctival SDB
- close the skin SDB
- palliate SDB of the external canthal ligament by lower eyelid support procedures [98].

3.7- Complementary gestures :

The lacrimal duct may be affected during resection of a tumoral lesion. In carcinology, tear duct reconstruction is rarely indicated. Given the relatively high average age of patients, lacrimal duct resection is well tolerated, as lacrimal secretion becomes rarer with age. In the case of limited lesions, repair procedures involve simple approximation of the permeable segments, and in the case of extensive lesions, arterial or venous grafts or neighboring mucous flaps. In our department, whenever possible, we perform a mono- or bicanaliculonasal catheterization, which is left in place for 2 to 3 months to calibrate the lacrimal ducts. If this fails, the patient is referred for a bypass dacryorhinocystostomy.

4- Repair of labio-chin PDS :

The lips have a sphincter function and are a key element in facial expression and mimicry. Their reconstruction must meet two main requirements:

- Functionally, labial amplitude must be restored in both the vertical and horizontal planes, to ensure salivary continence, good occlusion and correct labial dynamics, respectively.
- Morphologically, the reconstruction must respect the proportion of labial tissues, the continuity of the cutaneous-mucosal line and the symmetry of the commissures.

During any labial repair, it is essential to characterize the SDB according to whether it is superficial or full-thickness, its location on the red and/or white areas, the proportion of SDB to the total labial volume, and the location of the commissures in relation to the SDB itself.

It is also essential to assess the condition and available skin capital of adjacent areas that may be harvested [1].

5.1- Repair of upper lip PDS :

The upper lip can be divided into two aesthetic subunits. The first is lateral, bounded medially by the outer edge of the philtrum, superiorly by the nasolabial fold and laterally by the nasolabial fold. The second is medial, formed by Cupid's bow and the philtral ridges.

Reconstruction must therefore take these sub-units into account, as well as the need to maintain symmetry at Cupid's bow to avoid distortion in relation to the base of the nose. In men, hairiness must be taken into account.

5.1.1- PDS repair of the upper white lip:

5.1.1.1- Directed wound healing:

This process, which can have the following indications :

- waiting for the definitive anatomopathological result after excision of a skin tumor
- the animal bite
- primary management of electrical burns [13].

5.1.1.2- Direct suture:

Some types of SDB, whether transfixing or not, are suitable for this procedure, notably low cutaneous SDB close to the mucocutaneous junction and less than 1.5 cm in size [101].

5.1.1.3- Skin grafting:

GPT, which is rarely used as a first-line procedure, can be performed with the aesthetic units of the lip in mind, in burns surgery or philtrum reconstruction.

Retro-auricular skin is preferred, followed by supra-clavicular skin [102].

5.1.1.4- Locoregional flaps:

These flaps allow closure of small SDBs.

5.1.1.4.1- Advancement and/or rotation flaps :

*5.1.1.4.1. a- **Webster advancement flap**:*

This flap is a good solution for repairing PDS of the paraphiltral lateral subunits.

In this case, don't hesitate to extend the PDS to the entire white paraphiltral labial subunit to improve the aesthetic result.

Technically, a peri-alar skin excision is required, as well as a juxta-commissural excision. A wide jugal detachment allows the cheek to be rolled up along the nostril wing [74].

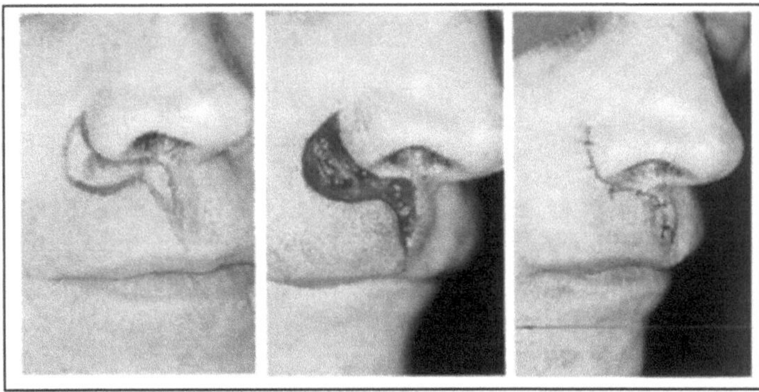

Figure 57: Webster nasolabial advancement flap

*5.1.1.4.1. b- **The nasolabial island flap** :*

This advancement-rotation flap, with a subcutaneous pedicle, is used for medium-sized defects near the junction of the nose wing and cheek. The lateral incision is placed along the nasolabial fold and the medial incision joins its apex on the nasolabial fold. It requires a detachment above the modiolus, which may be complicated by secondary retraction [103, 104].

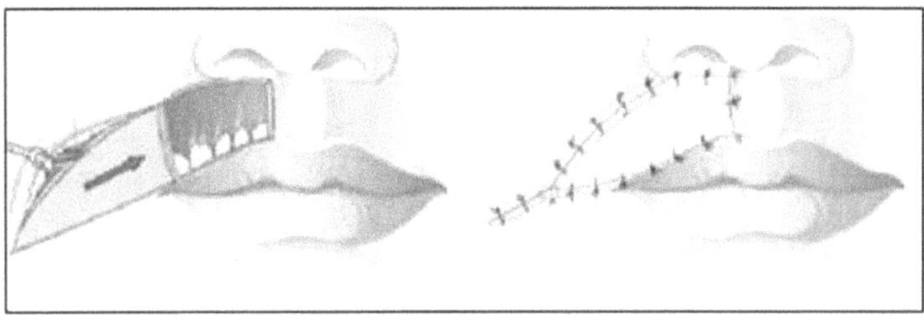

Figure 58: Islet nasolabial flap

*5.1.1.4.1. c- **Nasolabial flap with inferior pedicle :***

The use of a nasolabial flap with an inferior pedicle allows a fairly extensive reconstruction towards the medial part of the lip, with little scarring.

The superimposition of two inferior-pedicled nasolabial flaps allows the repair of total upper labial PDS, the Pierce procedure [26, 100].

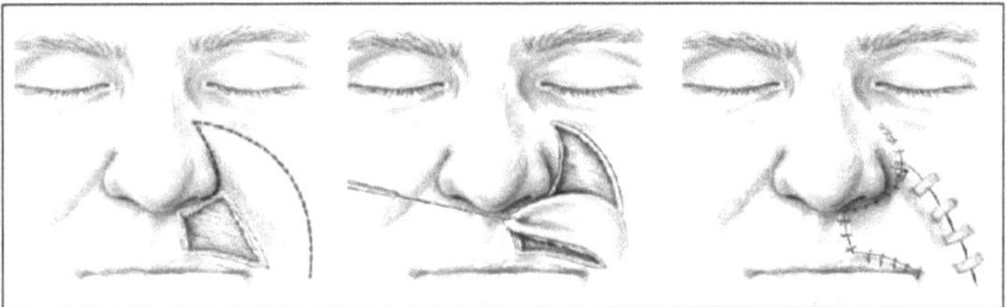

Figure 59: Nasolabial flap with inferior pedicle

*5.1.1.4.1. d- **The U-shaped jugal advancement flap :***

The cheek bordering the lip is an area of reparative skin reserve, enabling a U-shaped advancement flap to be used for extensive superficial SDB over three-quarters of the upper hemi-lip.

This flap requires a peri-alar crescent and a nostril anchor. The excess width of the flap is brought in for precise trimming at the inclination of the cutaneous-mucosal junction [105].

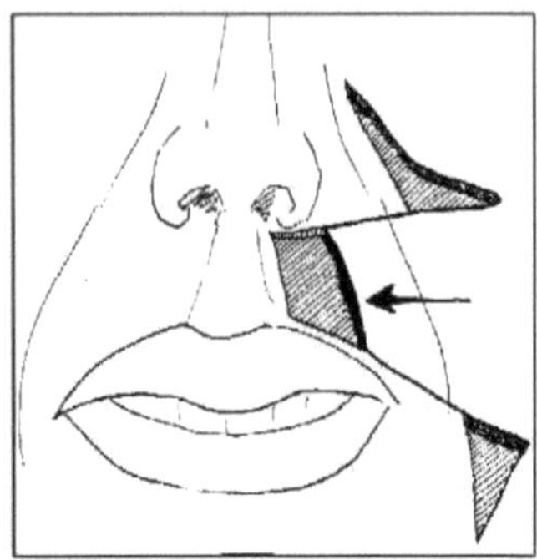

Figure 60: Préaux U-shaped jugal advancement flap

5.1.1.4.2- Transposition flaps:

They can be criticized for inducing asymmetrical displacements of remarkable lines or generating unsuitable scars.

5.1.2- PDS repair of the upper red lip:

We can sacrifice up to a third of the upper lip with first-line direct suture closure, especially in elderly subjects.

Apart from sutures, the various reconstruction objectives can only be achieved by using the buccal mucosa. While grafts are rarely indicated, multiple local flaps have been proposed, using the lip itself, the jugal mucosa and the tongue.

These flaps can be distributed according to the extent of the SDB.

5.1.2.1- SDB less than or equal to one-third of the upper lip:

5.1.2.1. a- <u>The Abbé flap</u> :

The abbot's flap is vascularized by the inferior coronary artery. It is a two-stage flap requiring secondary weaning of its pedicle.

Up to a third of the upper lip can be reconstructed, with the lower lip still flexible enough to give a quarter of its length without residual deformity.

This is a cutaneous-musculo-mucosal reconstruction. The width of the flap corresponds to the height of half of the upper lip's SDB.

The medial rotation point is based on the coronary artery, which must remain protected by the mucous membrane of the inner lip.

The flap is then rotated 180° and sutured plane by plane.

This Abbé flap gives good functional results. Aesthetic results are satisfactory, particularly for repairs of medial lesions where it reconstitutes the entire philtral aesthetic subunit [106, 107].

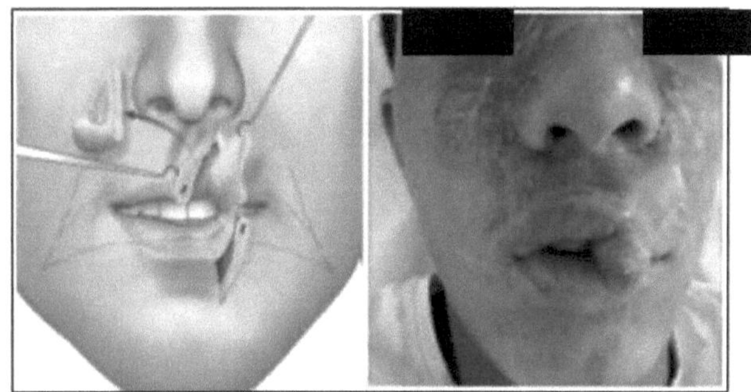

Figure 61: Abbot's flap in upper labial reconstruction

5.1.2.1. b- Estlander flap :

The Estlander flap, or full-thickness heterolabial rotation flap, uses the same principle as the Abbé flap for lateral juxta-commissural repair. It is also known as the Abbé-Estlander flap.

On the other hand, the commissural junction loses its naturally acute angle, to the benefit of an unsightly "rounded" effect of the neo-commissure. Secondary aesthetic correction by commissuroplasty is required.

On the one hand, it improves cosmetic appearance and, on the other, limits the microstomy effect [107].

5.1.2.2- DBP greater than one-third of the upper lip:

These SDBs require locoregional flaps to be taken from the cheek.

*5.1.2.2. a- **<u>Webster's jugal advancement flap</u>**:*

For SDB greater than half the upper lip, two cheek flaps are harvested with a crescent-shaped section of skin along the nostril wings.
Indications for this type of reconstruction are mainly reserved for paramedian PDS of the upper lip.

For medial repair and equal lip length, a contralateral Abbe flap is often used to recreate the aesthetic philtral subunit.
Unfortunately, this technique results in a receding upper lip with a microstomy and modification of the labial commissures [108, 109].

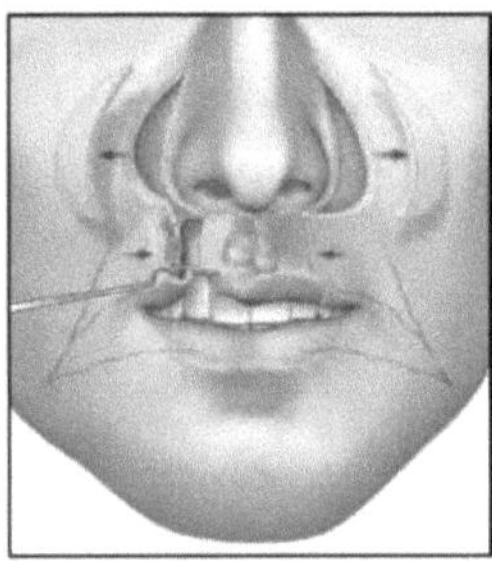

Figure 62: Jugal advancement flap for reconstruction of a paramedian PDS of the upper red lip

5.1.2.2. b- <u>Gillies fan flap</u>:

This is a flap taken around the nostril orifice, providing enough tissue to reconstruct an entire lip. The flap is cut to full thickness, including the mucosa, except at the commissural base, where the vascular pedicles must be respected.
Results are never very good, either functionally or aesthetically [105].

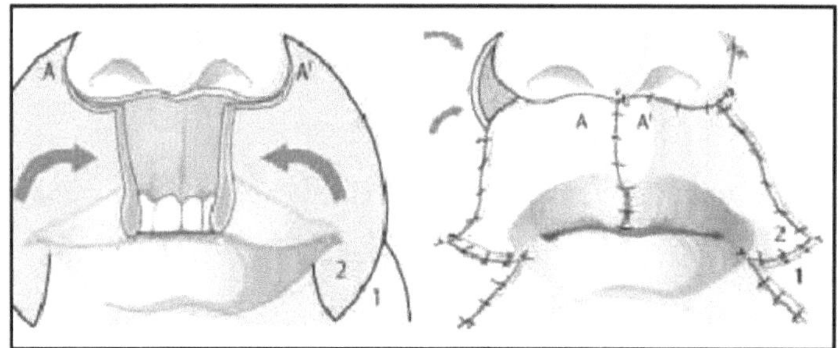

Figure 63: Gillies fan-shaped flap

5.1.2.2. c- Inverted Karapandzic flap :

Classically used to reconstruct the lower lip, this flap can also be used for large upper lip reconstructions.

The incision is pericommissural and concave medially. The flap is detached, preserving the vascular pedicles. There are two disadvantages: microstomia with labial incontinence and commissural displacement [108].

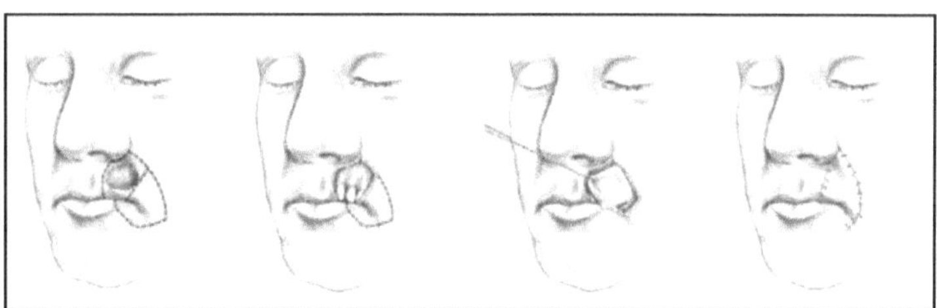
Figure 64: Inverted Karapandzic flap

5.1- Repair of lower lip PDS:

PDS of the lower lip are by far the most common to repair.

5.1.1- PDS repair of the lower white lip:

Lower white lip SDB repair problems are rarely isolated, and are far less complex in nature than those of the upper white lip, due to the absence of a structure equivalent to the philtrum.

5.1.1.1- Direct suture:

Whenever possible, direct suturing is the solution of choice. The axis of the spindle should be vertical. The maximum width is 1 cm [101].

5.1.1.2- Total skin grafting :

GPT can produce remarkable results in women with a light phototype when it respects the aesthetic subunits [109].

When it involves a lower hemi-lip, it must be sutured in w on the midline, the labiomental fold and the cutaneous-mucosal junction.

5.1.1.3- Locoregional flaps:

5.1.1.3. a- __Jugal advancement flap__ :

It is indicated for the repair of medial PDS of the lower white lip and chin.

The incision is made along the mucocutaneous junction and the basilar margin adjacent to the SDB [100].

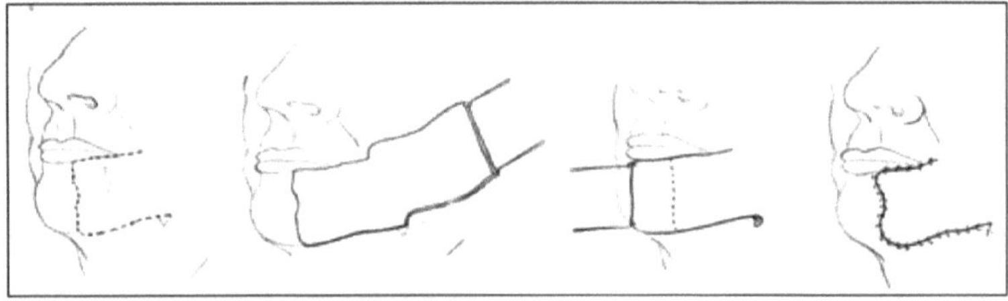

Figure 65: Jugal advancement flap for repair of the lower white lip

5.1.1.3. b- __Nasolabial flap with inferior pedicle__ :

This transposition flap is raised in the premuscular plane, with the inferior branch of the facial nerve preserved.

This technique gives good results, but there is a tendency towards a "pin cushion" appearance, which may require revision surgery [106].

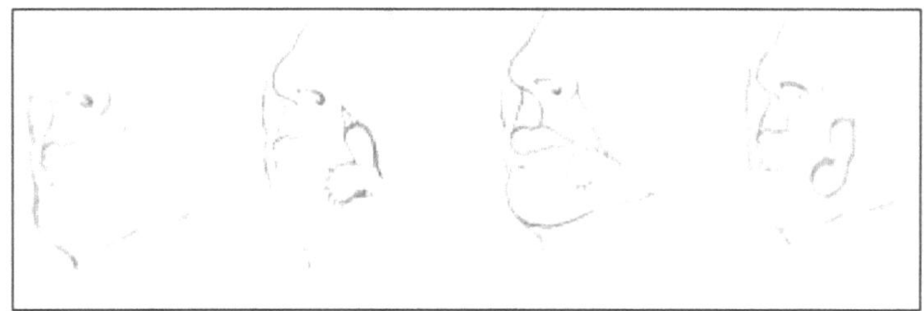

Figure 66: Nasolabial flap with inferior pedicle for repair of the lower white lip

5.1.1.3. *c- **Advancement autoplasty using the Burow technique :***

The Burow technique involves advancing a para-chin flap after excision of a nasolabial triangle.

It is intended for cutaneous SDB in the lower lateral aesthetic unit, in the shape of an isosceles triangle with a superior base. Its major drawback is commissural deformity [26].

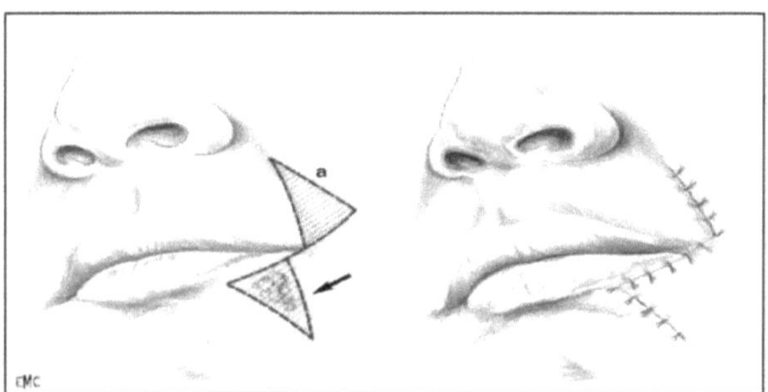

Figure 67: Advancement autoplasty using the Burow technique

5.1.2- PDS repair of the lower red lip:

In lower lip reconstruction, the rule of thirds can be applied schematically.

5.1.2.1- SDB less than or equal to one-third of the lower lip:

This is the indication for direct V or W sutures.

The repair is performed plane by plane, and the labio-cutaneous line must be anatomical. The V-shaped suture can be replaced by a W-shaped resection, which leaves a shorter scar [106].

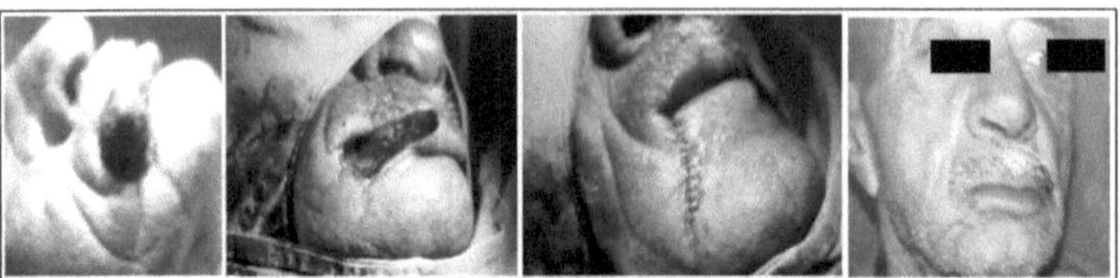

Figure 68: Direct suture of an inferior labial PDS

5.1.2.2- SDB between one-third and two-thirds of the lip lower :

For these SDBs, locoregional flaps taken from the contralateral lip are the solution.

5.1.2.2. a- Abbé-Estlander heterolabial flaps:

The Estlander procedure, already described, is aimed at lateral and juxta-commissural SDB [101, 109].

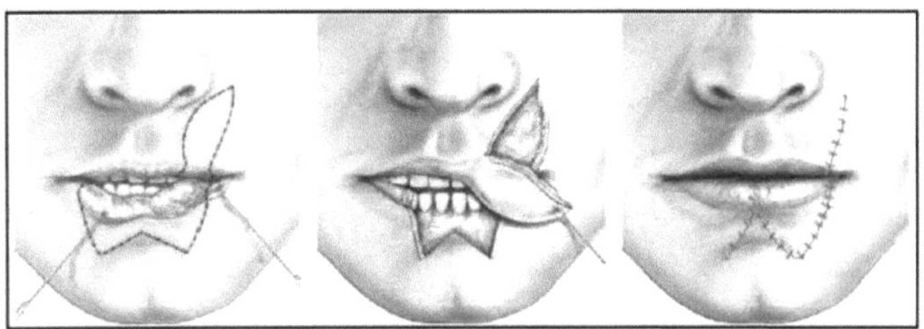

Figure 69: Abbe-Estlander heterolabial flaps

5.1.2.2. b- Johanson's staircase process :

This technique is interesting for lateral and juxta-commissural SDB, as the orbicular sphincter is preserved. It can also be used twice for medial SDB.

Removal of the tumor lesion results in a rectangular SDB. Lateral staircase incisions are made. Their length corresponds to half the length of the SDB.

The incision on each step is transfixing, allowing easy advancement. The lateral incision of the last step is concealed in the labiomental fold. Johanson's technique thus preserves sphincter function and lip vascularization. However, microstomy may be observed in half-lip resections [101, 108].

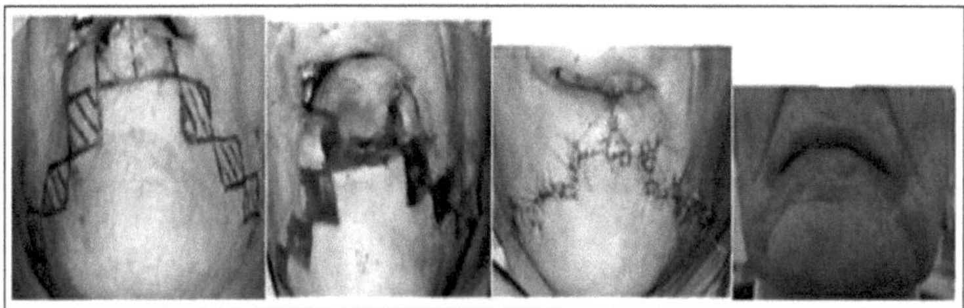

Figure 70: Johanson staircase process

*5.1.2.2. c- **<u>The Gillies fan flap</u>** :*

This flap enables reconstruction of a hemi-lip with the healthy juxta-commissural lip. Used bilaterally, it can be used to reconstruct an entire lip. Cut to full thickness, its displacement is improved by a *back cut.* It uses the tissue reserve of the commissural region and is deployed around it like a fan. It induces a relative microstomy, especially when used bilaterally. It does not reconstruct the red lip, but a mucosal or even tongue flap may be associated [109].

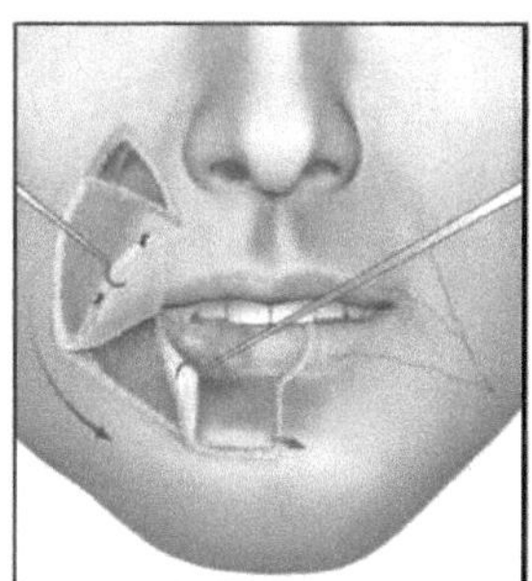

Figure 71: Gillies fan-shaped flap

5.1.2.3- SDB greater than two-thirds of the lower lip:

Two main techniques are mainly used for this type of delicate reconstruction, given the loss of sphincter function of the lip:

5.1.2.3. *a- __Camille Bernard flap__:*

The original technique, described by Camille Bernard, involves repairing the entire lower lip with two cheek advancement flaps. Cutaneous resection of the two commissural triangles with lower bases enables lateral labio-chin margin slippage. Each base is equal to half the labial DBP.

A triangular mucosal flap is then taken from the inner cheek. This flap is turned over, everted and sutured to the base of the skin resection triangle, thus reconstituting a new red lip.

The functional results of this technique are poor, with receding lower lip, poor occlusion and salivary leakage [108, 110].

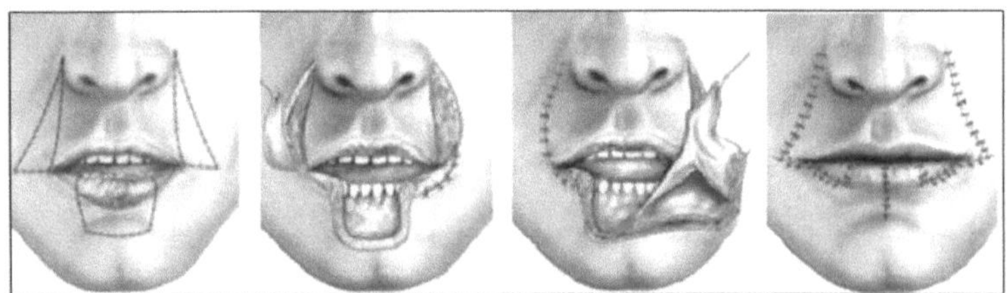

Figure 72: Camille Bernard flap

5.1.2.3. *b- __Webster's modified Camille Bernard flap__:*

Webster creates four offloading skin flaps, two in the nasolabial folds and two in the labiomental folds along the contour of the chin. This allows the flaps to advance more easily.

Reconstruction of the inferior vermilion can be performed using either mucosal flaps from the inner cheek or a tongue flap [111].

Reconstruction using this technique leads to better functional results than with the basic Camille Bernard technique. Nevertheless, there may still be imperfect lip continence due to the significant recession of the lower lip and the advancement of the upper lip.

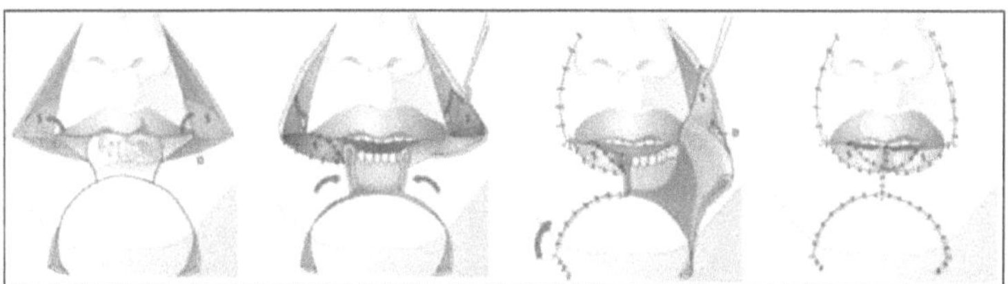

Figure 73: Camille Bernard flap modified by Webster

5.1.2.3. *c- **<u>Karapandzic flap</u>**:*

The principle is to take a cheek advancement flap with a superior base.

In this respect, it is similar to Gillies' fan-shaped flap, but the incision is not transfixing and preserves the mucosa.

The skin incision is arched concavely inwards. It begins at the base of the rheumatic spine and ascends towards the base of the nose, keeping clear of the labial commissure.

The vessels are dissected and respected. The mucosa of the cheek is respected, except for the first two centimetres to allow better advancement of the flap. The flap is then advanced and sutured to fill the SDB.

This technique allows reconstruction with continuous, sensitive lips, but often with a microstomy [112, 113].

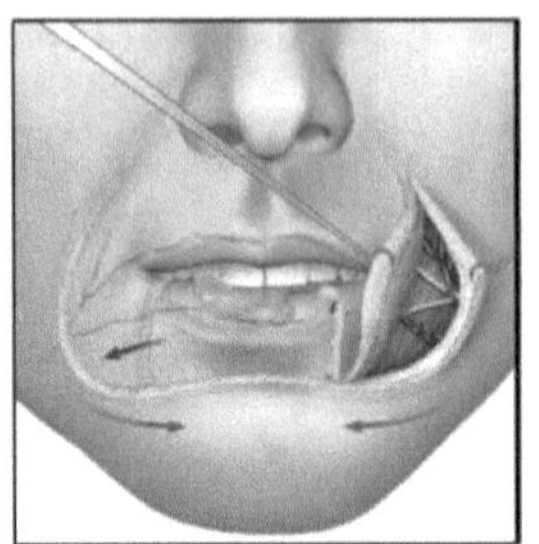

Figure 74: Karapandzic technique

5.2 Chin repair :

In addition to direct suturing, repair of SDB limited to this region can involve locoregional flaps, the most useful of which are the jugal advancement flap and the submental flap already described.

Conclusion

Reconstructive surgery of the face and neck offers a wide range of therapeutic techniques that have continued to develop over the years.

Loss of substance of the cephalic extremity can be secondary to multiple iatrogenic aggressions. Removal of skin tumors is the main cause. Reconstruction of these losses of substance can pose a number of difficulties for the surgeon, due to their extent and proximity to periorificial areas.

Choosing the most appropriate repair procedure is a fundamental step, requiring careful study of the specific features of the region to be repaired, the semiological characteristics of the loss of substance to be filled and the patient's background. The aim is to achieve the best possible functional and aesthetic result.

References

1. Huguier V, Dagrégorio G, Darsonval V, Arnaud D, Potier B, Rousseau P. Jugal reconstruction. Annales de chirurgie plastique esthétique, (2013)58; 457-514.

2. Albert S, Guedon C. Reconstructive surgery using micro-anastomosed flaps in cervicofacial carcinology. La lettre du cancérologue, (2011)20 ; 116-119.

3. Bédane C. Cutaneous tumors and their treatment. Annales de dermatologie et de vénérologie, (2016)143; 29.Bach C, Sannajust JP, Dehesdi D. Scars, scarring, directed healing, dressings and treatment of sequelae. Restorative surgery of the face and neck - volume 1. Surgical techniques. Chirurgie plastique et esthétique, 2011 ; 42-46.

4. Chavoin JP, Gangloff D. Grafting, flaps and expansion. Chirurgie plastique et esthétique, 2009 ; 18-38.

5. Lasurdy J. Management of palpebral tumors: general considerations. Journal français d'ophtalmologie, 2011 ; 741-754.

6. Jourdain A, Vimont T, Arnaud D, Darsonval V, Huguier V, Rousseau P. Reconstruction of superficial loss of substance of the nose. Annales de chirurgie plastique esthétique, (2013)58; 515-545.

7. Darsonval V, Arnaud D, Duron JB, Bardot J, Rousseau P. Full-thickness reconstruction of the nasal pyramid. Annals of aesthetic plastic surgery, (2013)58; 544-600.

8. Petit A, Boccara D, Caouat M, Mimoun M. Reconstruction of transfixing loss of substance of the nasal wing by contralateral nostril composite graft: about three cases. Annales de chirurgie plastique esthétique, (2013)59; 280-286.

9. Bessède JP. Lambeaux cutanés. Chirurgie plastique réparatrice de la face

et du cou : vol 1. Paris : Elsevier Masson ; 2011 p 84-97.

10. Revol M, Servant JM. Reconstruction of the nose. Manuel de chirurgie plastique reconstructrice et esthétique, 1993 ; 333-403.

11. Starkman SJ, Williams CT, Sherris DA. Flap Basics I: Rotation and Transposition Flaps. Facial Plast Surg Clin North Am. 2017 Aug;25(3):313-321. doi: 10.1016/j.fsc.2017.03.004. Epub 2017 May 30.
12. Amici JM, Dordain-Bigot ML, Wetterwal E, Bailly JY. Tissue motion analysis and flap principles. Chirurgie dermatologique, 2012; 131-144.
13. Bach CA, Wagner I, Lachiver X, Guth A, Baglin AC, Chabolle F. The free thoracodorsal performance flap in head and neck reconstructions. Annales françaises d'oto-rhino-laryngologie et de pathologie cervico-faciale, (2012)129; 192196.
14. Gao B, Xiao K, Zhu H, Sheng L, Yu Q, Mao X et al. An algorithm for using expanded cervical flaps to resurface facial defects based on five different methods. Burns, (2016)42; 1867-1874.
15. Eid IN, Arosarena OA. Reconstruction of cutaneous cancer defects in the head and neck.Otolaryngologic clinics of north America. 2021 (54), 379-395.
16. Cox A, Fort M. Nasal Reconstruction Involving Multiple Subunit Defects. Facial Plast Surg. 2017 Feb;33(1):58-66.
17. Amici JM, Cogrel O, Billy JY. Nose surgery. Chirurgie dermatologique, 2012; 181-195.
18. Derhy Y. Aesthetic reconstructive nose surgery. Medical publication, 2009; 7 pages.
19. Ian M, Jemery Bordeaux MD, MPH. Post-skin cancer alar reconstruction. Facial plastic surgery, (2013)29; 351-364.

20. Stigall L, Zitelli J. Reconstructing the nasal tips. British journal of dermatology, (2014)171; 23-28.

21. Chavoin JP, Grrido-Stowhas I. Chirurgie plastique et esthétique, 2009; 68-84.

22. Guillot P. Islet flaps: introduction, theoretical notions. Annals of dermatology and venereology, (2014)141; 10-11.

23. Lebas D. Islet flaps in the mediofacial setting. Annals of dermatology and venereology, (2014)141; 11.

24. Amici JM, Cogrel O, Bailly JY, Skaria AM. Nose surgery. Dermatologic surgery. 2017, 183-202.

25. Girijala RL, Ramamurthi A, Walker GD, Housewright C. Revisiting the Rintala advancement flap for nasal tip reconstruction. Dermatol Online J. 2020 Aug 15;26(8):13030/qt5dv0s7zx.

26. Bulai Livideanu C, Guillot P. Bilobed flap for repair of nasal loss of substance. Annals of dermatology and venereology, (2013)140; 191-192.

27. James BL. The physiology and biomechanics of skin flap. Facial plastic surgery clinics of north America. 2017 (25), 303-311.

28. Bailly JY. From hatchet flap to Rieger's hamlet. Annals of dermatology and venereology, (2012)139; 16-17.

29. Ettalbi S, Droussi H, Ouahbi S, Ibnouzahir M, Boubind EH. LLL plasty: a simple method for covering skin loss of substance. Annales de chirurgie plastique esthétique, (2013)58; 367-372.

30. Droussi H, Najeb Y. Dufourmentel's L-shaped flap for rhombus (LLL) to cover loss of cutaneous substance: 30 cases. Thesis 2009. Faculté de Médecine et de Pharmacie de Marrakech, 2009; 4 pages.

31. Amici JM. Nasal tip: unit repairs, uni and bilobed flaps. Annals of dermatology and venereology, (2015)142; 138-139.

32. Viniculllo C. Reconstructing the nasal dorsum. British journal of

dermatology, (2014)171; 7-16.

33. Dordain-Bigot ML. Repair of nasal tip loss of substance by Rieger flap. Annals of dermatology and venereology, (2012)139; 18-19.

34. Johnson TM, Swanson NA, Baker SR, Brown MD, Nelson BR. The Rieger flap for nasal reconstruction. Arch Otolaryngol Head Neck Surg. 1995 Jun;121(6):634-7.

35. Chaput B, Lauwers F, Lopez R, Saboye J, André A, Grolleau JL et al. Surgical anatomy of the nose in six aesthetic subunits. Annales de chirurgie plastique esthétique, (2013)58; 132-145.

36. Jourdain A. Superficial nasal reconstructions. Reconstructive surgery of the face and neck - volume 1. Surgical techniques. Chirurgie plastique et esthétique, 2011; 156-170.

37. Abbou R, Meningaud JP, Bosc R, Hersant B, Zemerline A, Baratte A. Superior pedicle nasolabial flap: towards improved surgical technique. Revue de stomatologie et de chirurgie maxillo-faciale, 2014; 1-5.

38. Cook JL. The reconstruction of nasal ala with interpolated flap from the cheek and forehead. British journal of dermatology, (2014)171; 29-36.

39. Abbou R, Meningaud JP, Bosc R, Hersant B, Zemirline A, Baratte A. Upper nasolabial flap, improving the surgical technique. Rev Stomatol Chir Maxillofac Chir Orale. 2014 Dec;115(6):361-5. doi: 10.1016/j.revsto.2014.06.004. Epub 2014 Jul 16.

40. Cogrel O. Burget transient superior pedicle nasolabial flap. Annals of dermatology and venereology, (2014)141; 24.

41. Cante V, Cogrel O. Burget transient superior pedicle nasolabial flap: a technique suitable for nasal tip reconstruction, about five cases. Annals of Dermatology and Venereology, (2011)138; 194.

42. Bouhanna A, Bruant-Rodier C, Himu S, Talmant JC, Bollecker V, Glicksman J. Reconstruction of the nostril wing by Burget superior

pedicle nasolabial flap: about seven cases. Annales de chirurgie plastique esthétique, (2009)53 ; 272-277.

43. Salmon PJM. Repair of the nasal sidewall. British journal of dermatology, (2014)171; 17-22.

44. Cogrel O. Reconstruction of transfixing loss of substance of the nostril wing with a Pers turned island nasolabial flap. Annals of dermatology and venereology, (2015)142; 139-140.

45. Wiart T. The Pers flap. Annals of dermatology and venereology, (2015)142; 25.

46. Celerier C, Cristofari JP, Halimi C, Maubec E, Barry B, Albert S. Interest and indications of the forehead flap in nasal loss of substance. Annales françaises d'oto-rhino-laryngologie et de pathologie cervico-faciale, (2013)130; 57.

47. Rayan JS, Melvyn S, David-Kim D. Paramedian forehead flap. Oral maxilla-facial surgery clincs, (2014)26; 401-410.

48. Fisher H, MD. Nasal reconstruction with the paramedian forehead flap: details for success. Facial plastic surgery, (2014)30; 318-331.

49. Kendler M, Averbeck M, Wetzig T. Reconstruction of nasal defects with forehead flaps in patients older than 75 years of age. Journal of the European academy of dermatology and venereology, (2014)28; 662-666.

50. Faris C, Erden PV, Vuyk H. The midline central artery forehead flap. JAMA facial plastic surgery, (2015)17; 16-22.

51. Stephen S, Park MD. The single stage forehead flap in nasal reconstruction. Archives of facial plastic surgery, 2002; 32-36.

52. Ozdemir R, Sungur N, Sensoz O. Reconstruction of facial defects with superficial temporal artery island flaps. Plastic reconstructive surgery, 2002.

53. Arnaud D, Potier B, Jeufroy C, Darsonval V, Rousseau P. The Schmid-

Meyer frontotemporal flap in nasal reconstructions. Revue de stomatologie et de chirurgie maxillofaciale, (2012)113 ; 423-432.

54. Han Y, Ai Y, Lei Y, Yang L, Zhang H. Reconstruction of partial nose defects with retro-auricular free flap transplantation. Zhonghua Zheng Xing Wai Ke Za Zhi, (2002)18; 204-205.

55. Guillot P. Cheek surgery. In: Amici JM. Chirurgie dermatologique. Paris : Elsevier Masson ; 2012 p 217-23.

56. Pepper JP, Shan R. Local flaps: cheek and lip reconstruction. JAMA Fac Plast Surg. 2013; 15: 374-82.

57. Jourdain A. Cheek reconstruction. Plastic reconstructive surgery of the face and neck: vol 1. Paris : Elsevier Masson ; 2011 p 192-9.

58. Pontes L, Ribeiro M, Vrancks JJ, Guimaraes J. The new bilaterally pedicled V-Y advancement flap for facial reconstruction. Plastic surgery unit, Portuguese institute of oncology, (2001)109; 1870-1874.

59. Erden VD, Paul A, Peter JFM. Secondary intention healing after excision of nonmelanoma skin cancer of the head and neck: static evaluation of prognostic values of wound characteristics and final cosmetic results. Plastic and reconstructive surgery, Journal of the American society of plastic surgeon, (2008)122; 1747-1755.

60. Rapstine ED, Knaus WJ, Thornton JF. Simplifying cheek reconstruction: a review of over 400 cases. Plastic and reconstructive surgery. Journal of the American society of plastic surgeons (2012)129; 1291-1299.

61. Bailly JY. White upper lip repair. The dermatologist's point of view. Annals of dermatology and venereology, (2015)142; 324-325.

62. Yenidunya MO, Demirseren ME, Ceran C. Bilobed flap reconstruction in infraorbital skin defects. Plastic and reconstructive surgery. Journal of the American society of plastic surgeons, 2007; 145-150.

63. Cass ND, Terella AM. Reconstruction of the cheek. Facial Plast Surg

Clin North Am. 2019 Feb ; 27(1) :55-56.

64. Habib F. Two-stage surgery of an aggressive temporal carcinoma with jugal advancement-rotation plasty repair. Annals of dermatology and venereology, (2013)140; 181-182.

65. Wiart T. Repair of loss of substance in the jugopalpebral region by two jugal and palpebral advancement-rotation flaps. Annals of dermatology and venereology, (2012)139; 91-92.

66. Lebas D, Wiart T Modiano P. Jugonasal basal cell carcinoma: repair by jugal advancement flap. Annals of dermatology and venereology, (2012)139; 83.

67. Baraer F, Loze S, Duteille F, Pannier M, Darsonval V. The orbito-nasogeal flap: anatomical and technical study. Annales de chirurgie plastique esthétique, (2005)50; 288-295.

68. Caquant L, Mojallal A, Collin AC, Bouletreau P, Breton P. Jugal reconstruction by vertical translation flap. Revue de stomatologie et de chirurgie maxillofaciale, (2008)109; 15-19.

69. Zweteyenga N, Lutz JC, Vidal N, El Bouihi M, Siberchicot F, Martin D. The pedicled submental flap. Revue de stomatologie et de chirurgie maxillofaciale, (2007)108 ; 210-214.

70. Klinic H, Geyik Y, aytekin AH. Double skin paddled superficial temporofascial flap for the reconstruction of full-thickness cheek defects. The journal of craniofacial surgery, (2013)24; 92-95.

71. Sinna R, Qassemyar Q. The thoracodorsal perforator flap. Annales de chirurgie plastique esthétique, (2011)56 ; 142-148.

72. Perignon D, Qassemyar Q, Benhaim T, Robbe M, Delay E, Sinna R. From Tansini to Angrigiani: Improvements and refinements of the thoracodorsal flap. Annales de chirurgie plastique esthétique, (2011)56;

149-155.

73. Minoun M, Boccara D, Chaouat M. Skin expansion and repair of burn sequelae. Annales de chirurgie plastique esthétique, (2011)56; 358-368.
74. Arnaud D, Beuzeboc M, Huguier V, Darsonval V, Rousseau P. Aesthetic frontotemporal reconstruction. Annales de chirurgie plastique esthétique, (2013)58; 389-427.
75. Egasse D. Surgery of the forehead and eyebrow region. Chirurgie dermatologique, 2012; 145-155.
76. Beauvillain de Montreuil C, Malard O. Forehead and temple repairs. Restorative surgery of the face and neck - volume 1. Techniques chirurgicales - Chirurgie plastique et esthétique, 2011 ; 201-210.
77. Pepper JP, Shan R. Local flaps: cheek and lip reconstruction. JAMA facial plastic surgery, (2013)15; 374-382.
78. Sharma RK, Makkar S, Parashar A, Tuli P. Frontal reconstruction with frontal musculocutaneous V-Y Island flaps. Journal of the American society of plastic surgeons, 2008; 1855-1873.
79. Hussain W, Hafij J, Salmon P. Frontalis-based pedicle flaps for the single-stage repair of large defects of the forehead and frontal scalp. Dermatological surgery and lasers. British journal of dermatology, (2012); 771-774.
80. Egasse D. Surgery of the temporal region. In: Amici JM. Chirurgie dermatologique, 2012; 157-163.
81. Igde M, Yilanci S, Bali YY, Unlu E, Duzgun S, Pekdemir I. Reconstruction of tissue defects developing after excision of non-melanoma malignant skin-tumor in scalp and forehead regions. Turk neurosurgery, (2015)25; 888-894.
82. Redondo P. Simplifying forehead and temple reconstruction: A narrative

review. J. Clin. Med. 2023, 12(16), 5399

83. Voilliot C, Truchtet F, Pouaha J. Basal cell carcinoma of the temporal region, anterior pedicle transposition flap repair. Annals of dermatology and venereology, (2014)141; 51-52.

84. Foyatier JL, Voulliaume D, Brun A, Dionyssopoulos A. Surgical treatment of facial burn sequelae. Annales de chirurgie plastique esthétique, (2011)56 ; 388-407.

85. Bruneau S, Arnaud D, Rousseau P, Belmahi A, Duron JB, Gray-Bobo A et al. Aesthetic aspects of eyelid reconstruction. Annales de chirurgie plastique esthétique, (2013)58; 437-456.

86. Secchi T. Is direct suturing suitable for supra-centimeter palpebral and subpalpebral loss of substance. Annals of dermatology and venereology, (2012)139; 88.

87. Epinoza GM, Prost am. Upper eyelid reconstruction. Facial plastic surgery clinics, (2016)24; 173-182.

88. Robert M, Rousseau P, Arnaud D, Potier B, Hu W, Darsonval V. Reconstruction of the external canthus by tarso-conjunctival transposition flaps and Hübner grafts. Annales de chirurgie plastique esthétique, (2014)59; 287-293.

89. Galatoire O, Zmuda M. Palpebral reconstruction. Eye surgery. Société Française d'Ophtalmologie, 2016; 43-69.

90. Echchaoui A, Ben Yachou M, Houssa A, Kajout M, Oufkir AA, Hajji C et al. Management of eyelid carcinomas: a retrospective bi-centric study of 64 cases. French Journal of Ophthalmology, (2016)39; 187-194.

91. Cogrel O. Excision of a Dubreuilh melanoma in situ of the lower palpebral region and reconstruction with a Mustardé flap. Annals of dermatology and venereology, (2016)143; 167-168.

92. Adenis JP, Camezind P, Robert PY. Eyelid reconstructive surgery. Restorative surgery of the face and neck - volume 1. Techniques chirurgicales - Chirurgie plastique et esthétique, 2011 ; 176-189.
93. Blatière V. Eyelid surgery. Chirurgie dermatologique, 2012; 165-180.
94. Holds JB. Lower eyelid reconstruction. Facial plastic surgery clinics, (2016)24; 183191.
95. Chavoin JP. Eyelids. Chirurgie plastique et esthétique, 2009; 53-59.
96. Machado WL, Gurfinkel PC, Gualberto GV, Sanpaio FM, Treu CM. Modified tripier flap in reconstruction of lower eyelid. Anais Brasileiros de dermatologia, (2015)90; 108-110.
97. Bardot J, Casanova D, Malet T. Reconstructive eyelid surgery. EMC-chirurgie, (2004)1; 365-390.
98. Belmajdoub M, Jacomet PV, Benillouche P, Galatoire O. Upper palpebral reconstruction using the Cutler-Beard method: retrospective evaluation of 16 cases. French Journal of Ophthalmology, (2015)38; 607-614.
99. Bessède JP. Reconstructive surgery of the lips. Reconstructive surgery of the face and neck - volume 1. Techniques chirurgicales - Chirurgie plastique et esthétique, 2011 ; 212226.
100. Lubek JE, Ord RA. Lip reconstruction. Oral maxillofacial surgery clinics, (2013)25; 203-214.
101. Beltramina G, Kadheb N, Cassier S, Costantinescu G, Vazquez MP, Picard A. Cutaneous-mucosal composite graft for labial reconstruction of bite loss. Annales de chirurgie plastique esthétique, (2012) 57; 292-295.
102. Egasse D. Surgery of the lower lip, the dermatologist's point of view Annales de dermatologie et de vénéréologie, (2015)142; 325.

103. Kaufman AJ. Surgical gem: Island advancement flaps for lip reconstruction. Australian journal of dermatology, (2014)55; 201-203.

104. Bailly JY. Surgery of the lips. Chirurgie dermatologique, 2012; 197-209.

105. Rousseau P, Arnaud D, Huguier V, Chemli H, Dhouib M, Bali D et al. Restorative and aesthetic lip surgery. Annals of aesthetic plastic surgery, (2013)58; 601-627.

106. Kumar A, Shetty PM, Bhambar RS, Gattumeedhi SR, Kumar RM, Kumar H. Versatility of Abbe-Estlander flap in lip reconstruction. Journal of clinical and diagnostic research, (2014)8; 18-21.

107. Malard O, Corre P, Durand N, Dréno B, Beauvillain C, Espitalier F. Surgical repair of labial loss of substance. Annales françaises d'oto-rhino-laryngologie et de pathologie cervico-faciale, (2010)127 ; 58-72.

108. Chavoin JP, Garrido I. Lips. Chirurgie plastique et esthétique, 2009 ; 89-97.

109. Huguier V, Bertheuil N, Parry F, Robiolle C, Dagrégorio G. Posttraumatic reconstruction of the lower lip after total or subtotal amputation using the Camille-Bernard technique modified by Webster. Annales de chirurgie plastique esthétique, (2013)58; 166-174.

110. Brinca A, Vieiraa R, Andrade P, Figueiredo A. Karapandzic flap and Bernard-Burrow- Webster flap for reconstruction of the lower lip. Anais Brasileiros de dermatologia, (2011)86; 156-159.

111. Espitalier F, Rouger A, Philippe Y, Dréno B, Malard O. Reconstruction of the lower lip using the Karapandzic technique. Annales françaises d'oto-rhino- laryngologie et de chirurgie cervico-faciale, (2012)129; 42.

112. Azevedo DM, Nagassaki E, De Carvalho AS, Secco Lafayette KA, Gonzalez E, Saldanha OR et al. Lower lip reconstruction using the Karapandzic technique. Brazilian journal of plastic surgery, (2013)28; 168-171.

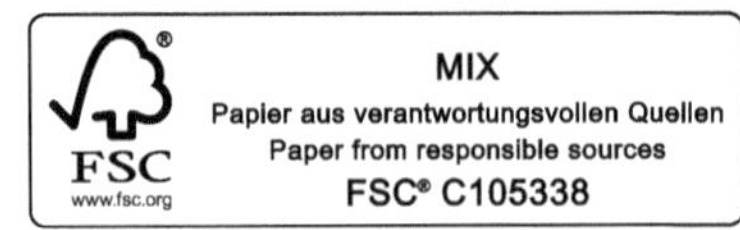

Printed by Books on Demand GmbH, Norderstedt / Germany